The Echo of a Footfall

The
Echo
of a
Footfall

Patricia Scampion

Matador
9 Priory Business Park,
Wistow Road, Kibworth Beauchamp,
Leicestershire. LE8 0RX
Tel: 0116 279 2299
Email: books@troubador.co.uk
Web: www.troubador.co.uk/matador
Twitter: @matadorbooks

ISBN 978 1838591 724

British Library Cataloguing in Publication Data.
A catalogue record for this book is available from the British Library.

Printed and bound in Great Britain by 4edge Limited
Typeset in 12pt Adobe Jenson Pro by Troubador Publishing Ltd, Leicester, UK

Matador is an imprint of Troubador Publishing Ltd

For Claire and Helen

Part I

Asylum

I

1926

THE FLOOR WAS COLD AND THE BEDSTEAD hard as pokers that first day. I were sixteen and I'd birthed my baby not a three night before. They'd brought me there from the workhouse at the end of the day: my baby were snatched from me and they'd marched me, one on each arm, bumragged me, out of the room where I'd borne him. My belly ached and I were bleeding; I was crying and I couldna' see for the tears in me eyes. I kept asking for them to give him back, to let 'im suckle; but they brought me here and laid me on a bed, and told me to keep quiet or I'd waken them ladies in t' other beds. And my chest was worst: hot and swollen, and tingling with sharp needle points when the milk came. I just wanted my baby. I wanted to suckle him. They'd let me feed him after he were born, said it was good for him to have his ma's milk, and it had been sore painful, but so good to feel his little mouth searching for and suckin' on me. I wanted him back but they'd taken him from me. They said I couldna' care for him, though I told them me ma would help. But they said: now where was she gone, and

3

I didna' know. She'd taken me to workhouse when the pains started, but then they'd sent her away.

I lay on top o' bed all night, then in the morning I slid down behind and peeked out to see what was to do. But I were so cold. And I wanted to sleep an' all. I saw I was in a great room with a great high ceiling, like as I'd never seen before, and the sun were shinin' in through long, high windows, but it didna' warm me; and there were beds down both sides and a great many women getting up and dressing. They put on long woollen skirts, down to the floor, like as old biddies wear, 'n like as I'd not seen for years, and aprons and shawls, and some had shoes and some clogs and some ankle-Jacks, and they brushed each other's hair, and some of them didn't seem to know what to do and others cared for 'em. And they talked and sometimes they laughed, and I didna' think they saw me, so I stayed quiet. But I didna' want to be there, I didna', I didna'.

Then two of 'em came and told me, "Get dressed", and they left me some clothes, but I just stopped where I was and held on to the doll they gave me last night. He were wood with metal hooks to join his arms and legs, and he had a face painted on him as was wearing away so you could only see a bit o' his eyes. I didna' know when they gave him me, or why… perhaps it was when I wouldna' let go of my baby's blanket. I'd never had a doll like that before, not even when I were a wee little girl, but he gave me a bit o' comfort. Even the pain of his metal joints diggin' in me when I held him tight was a bit o' help, felt better than the pains in me belly and me chest: made me forget 'em a while.

Then the ladies all started to leave. I could hear the echoes of their feet out the door and down the stairs. Everything were echoing in here, voices, feet, and the laughing, jumpin' off the walls at you. And they were all hard sounds, like metal spoons in a drawer: nothing soft and comforting. Then, as they left, one of them came o'er to me. She bent over to look at me from under the end of the bed, and I wanted to laugh and cry, all at same time: she looked like an ole boggart with her head all upside down. But she looked kindly. I couldna' tell like that if she were old or young, but her hair were grey and pulled back from her face, and her eyes were grey as well, and soapy soft. I knew from her eyes she wouldna' hurt me. I wanted her not to hurt me, I couldna' be hurt no more, please.

"Sure, an' my name's Liza, Leeeeeza, mind, and not short for owt. 'Tis from the Russian. Call me by my name and I'll answer ye, but call me Elizabeth or some such nonsense and I'll not be for bothering. And will ye be comin' out o' there, so we can see what y're at?" I started crying again and the milk and the needles in my chest came, but mebbe she might help me, so I crawled out of my hidey-hole and stood up.

And she stood up as well, and she were taller than me and quite thin, and she frowned at me and mebbe she were cross, but she tut-tutted and reached out to stroke my cheek, ever so gentle.

"Jesus, Mary and Joseph, now what's a waif like you doing here? Come, come with me."

And she led me through a doorway to a row of white basins in the next room with taps above 'em, and she took the clothes off me as if I were a child. And I let her take 'em, and I let her wash me. I didna care: they'd done worse to me when the baby were comin'. Then she took the doll from me and found me rags for the bleeding, and she bound my chest with strips o' cloth, and I put on the fresh chemise she gave me, and a skirt like t' others.

Then she looked in my eyes and shook her head and gave me the doll back and led me back to my bed. "Now, go with the nurses: they're surely waiting for you. But stop." She caught my arm. "Be tellin' me your name first."

"'Tis Mary, Liza."

"Mother of God! Ye were well named. Another virgin birth, no doubt, and an Angel Gabriel wi' sovereigns in his pocket and idle promises on his lips. Go!"

And she were right: the nurses were waiting, though they looked to me just like t' other ladies, with their long skirts and their aprons, 'cept they had caps on their heads, and collars on their necks, and their aprons were starched stiff and shiny white. But they didn't smile. "Silly girl, you've missed your breakfast but you have to see the doctor this morning. Come with us. This way."

And Liza was gone, so what should I do?

One of them took my elbow and the other gave me a push in the middle o' me back, and they took me, so fast I couldna' keep up, out the door I'd come in through last night and down a flight of stone stairs to a long corridor with windows all along one side, high up so I couldna' see out, and then into a room wi' wood on all the walls, and benches round it, and a great polished wooden door. I were glad to get there for I were out o' breath and I kept trippin' on the hem o' me skirt. Then when the door opened they led me through it in front of a great desk, where a man, must've been the doctor, though I'd not ever seen a doctor before, was writing in a ledger, like the grocer totting the bill.

He didn't look up so all I could see were 'is balding head, his high starched collar, and his long fingers holding the pen. There was another woman in the room and without looking at me he waved his hand at her, and she shuffled me off to the side of the room and undressed me, pulling off the bindings as Liza had put on me with cold rough hands. She made me stand on the weighing scales. "Stand straight or I can't see how tall you are, and don't snivel."

I was cold and I felt shamed, standing naked holding the doll, with the step of the scales rattling as I shivered. But it

6

were worse when she took t' doll and led me back in front of the doctor.

Then he looked me up and down and turned me round, poked me and prodded me, and put tubes in his ears from like a trumpet he put on my chest, but he never ever looked in my eyes. It were discomfiting being looked at but yet not being looked at.

When he'd had enough of me, he started writing again, not stopping as he asked, "Name?"

"Mary, sir, Mary Pearson."

"How old are you, Pearson?" His voice was cold and 'ard and I was afeared.

"Sixteen, sir." I swallowed so as to try and stop me tears.

"And can you read and write?"

"No, sir."

He looked up, sighed, and turned to the nurse. "Moral defective. She has clearly just given birth and is underweight, but I see no sign of disease."

"She gave them trouble in the workhouse, sir. Mania, they thought. Couldn't control her. Wouldn't let go of her babe. They feared for its safety. And prattling all the time of her mother."

"Ah. Well, she's calm now. She needs to eat a healthy diet to fatten her up, to breathe fresh air and take some exercise, and, above all, she needs a sober Christian routine. Record any episodes of mania, and I will examine her again in six months. Fetch the next one for me to see."

"Please sir, c-c-can I not go home? My mother..."

"Get her dressed." He didn't even look at me this time. He turned back to his ledger and the nurse pulled me to the side of the room and gave me me clothes. I tried to escape her grip on my arm but I could not, and no-one took any note of my tears or words anyways. She gave me the bindings but I couldna' do them mesel', so I put them in me apron. Then they gave me the doll again, but he were no comfort, and someone took me back to Liza and the other ladies and told them to show me what I had to do.

After that, one day followed on another. There were a day bell rang when we had to rise in morning, and I watched t' other ladies to follow what they did. They all looked the same to me, and the nurses as well. And if I looked too much at them they turned their heads away or frowned at me, though I swear they looked more at me than I did at them. Only Liza spoke to me.

"What should I do, Liza? They watch me." I whispered so as they shouldn't hear.

"Take no notice. When they get used to you happen they'll stop staring."

"But I'm afeared of them, and I've got pinch marks on my arms from 'em from when they want me to move quick, like when we go for breakfast."

"That's the nurses as pinch you, and they'll nip your wrist or trip you up if you don't watch out, 'specially if it's a bad day for 'em. Just do as you're told."

"And I hate them breakfasts as well. I feel as I can't breathe with all that great number of women, all together in that great room. Liza, it's so big I can't see from one end to t' other, and they all bicker and mither and make such a noise."

"And their chatter echoes off the walls. For sure I understand ye. Even I would be for putting me hands over me ears. But you'll be getting used to it."

"And the porridge is thin and cold when we get it."

"Stop tha moaning. Beggars canna be choosers, and you're not for starvin'."

And I knew she were right. I weren't starving, I'd ate worse than this before.

After breakfast we'd all go back to our wards to tidy and clean. Then the Charge, for that's what they called her (she were like a chief nurse: she ordered the others around), she'd come and see our work. She'd run a finger over some tiles: "Nurse, when were these last damp-dusted?" Or she'd find the grate needed blacking, or the fire re-laying, though I never saw the ward fire lit in all the time I was there. There was always summat wrong, though we dusted and polished, mopped and scrubbed as hard as we could; emptied the night commodes (ugh, fow' task) and cleaned them, opened the tops of the windows so the smell went, and made the beds so the corners o' the sheets were folded just so.

"That's her job, to find fault," Liza laughed. "You wait till she brings the Visitors around, or Matron: *my nurses keep the ward perfect,* she'll tell them, *it's so important our ladies are set a good example.* Ha! Most of 'our ladies' have kept better houses than any of 'em."

"So, why are they here, Liza?"

"Sure, 'n you watch them and you'll see why. We're all mad, my dear, we're all mad. Lunatics, they say."

"So are you mad, Liza?"

"Happen I must be."

"But *I'm* not mad, Liza, I only had a baby."

"Shouldna' ha' done that, wi' out a man to speak for 'ee. Babes are the work of the Devil, Mary, and sure, the Devil's at work in here, you watch and you'll see."

"But I want to go home, Liza. I've work in a kitchen. Me ma will help me care for me baby. How can I get out?"

"Only the doctors can let you go. Tell that to them. And will y' be stoppin' plaguing me with questions."

So I did. I bit my tongue, and we went to the airing courts. Every day the nurses took us: down the stairs, along the corridor, our footsteps echoing so we sounded like a troop of pals from the Great War, marching through the streets. But *their* feet echoed off the back-to-backs, the homes they loved, ours were just thrown back at us by the shiny green tiles on the walls, like dropped coffin nails bouncing off a wareh'seman's floor, telling us not to dawdle. We'd pass the great clock on the wall, and sometimes you'd hear someone shouting or crying, but far away, or the slam of a door, or someone running, the echo of footsteps... and then we'd get to the open spaces: flower beds and paths and benches to sit on, but all still inside high walls. And there we'd have to get our "exercise".

The first time I went I just stood and looked up at the sky, and I could hear birds singing, and I cried, and I felt so tired I coulda' laid down and slept just for ever and ever. And I wanted my brother to be there: Tommy, where are you? You'd know what those birds were. You were always cleverer 'n me. Remember when you were five and I were seven and we used to run wild in the woods and the fields? You always knew how to get back to Auntie Nell, though she never cared where we were so long as we were back by nightfall. But we had to get back to baby Sam. Where are you both now? We were always together before she sent you away. I miss you, I miss you. And I miss my baby, I miss my baby so.

I looked to find Liza but she were away, walking along the path round the edge of the airing court, her head down. If she didn't want me, who else would? No-one, no-one cared. I were just alone. But then she were all I got, so I had to run to catch up with her. "Please, Liza, please. I need to find my baby, I need to, I need to. He's mine. He needs me. I want to hold him. I want to feed him. How can I get out of here?"

"Catch your breath and quiet down. Now be leavin' me alone, won't you. I've told 'ee: I have no time for babies. There's no way out of this place. If there's them that'll speak for thee outside..."

"My mother…"

"Mebbe the Devil has got her tongue as well."

"But, Liza, my baby…"

"I will NOT listen to talk of babies, I will not! Walk, or you'll catch your death of cold. But do not bother me with talk of babies."

And she took my arm and drew it through hers and patted my hand, but her face was all over stern and cross, and I dared not say else, so I faced into the wind and let it dry my tears, while we walked round and round. Back and forth we went, round and round, so many women. I watched. Some of them talked to themselves, some of them stared at me, some of them put their hands over their ears or shouted or laughed, but most just walked, shawls around their shoulders, hands 'neath their aprons for to keep 'em warm. Mebbe they were all shadows: black, long-skirted shadows. Perhaps they weren't real at all. Perhaps this were all just a bad dream, and I'd wake soon and I'd be in my attic bed beside me ma, ready for another day in the kitchens. But my baby was real, and I ached to the very bottom of my stomach for him, and my breasts ached to feed him, and then the needles came in my chest again and the warm wetness soaked through my chemise again, but I didn't dare tell Liza.

In the afternoons, after lunch in the great dining hall, we were taken to the airing courts again, but there were fewer of us as many of the women went off with the nurses. Liza said she were off to work in the sewing room and that others worked in the laundry or the kitchens. Then, when they came back, we had our supper and were in bed before you could say "Jack Robinson", and even before the sun went down. I would watch the shadows growing along the walls and wonder who put the flowers on the table at the end of the ward every day, big sunny yellow autumn blooms, like backyard chickens,

I thought, with their wings clipped, brightly feathered but hobbled, caught for ever in a cage, jumping at the light: like me, caged, but I were no good for owt now, even for layin'. And I'd fall asleep trying to stop out the sounds of the women in the other beds snoring and coughing, talking in their sleep, fidgeting and farting.

Some nights the shadows would grow so big and my bed were so small I'd think they'd carry me off: p'rhaps that's what they meant by the Valley of the Shadow of Death. P'rhaps I were going to die, p'rhaps that's what happened when they took a baby off you: you were locked away till you died. If this room were smaller I'd be safer, but as it grew darker it grew bigger and bigger...

Then one night I were woken. Someone was stood by my bed in the moonlight. She bent over me and put her hand 'neath my sheets reaching for me. Then she let her chemise fall off her, so she were standing with nowt on, in front of me, her breasts hanging low from her chest, like as they'd been pulled and stretched, and the skin on her belly wrinkled and sagging and marked with white scars. I thought I would scream but I opened my mouth and couldna' make a sound come out. I wasn't afeared of her nakedness: I'd seen women a' plenty undressed in the bath houses me ma had taken me, but she smiled, and her closeness, the sour smell of her body... and what would she do next? I feared she were going to climb into my bed, but then Liza appeared. She took the woman's hand and, picking up her chemise, led her back to her own bed. Then she came back to stroke the hair from my face. "Go to sleep now, she won't bother thee again tonight. That's Susan. She's harmless, just looking for a man to hold and warm her."

And I did go back to sleep, though my bed were not so safe now, and in the morning I looked for Susan. I saw the ladies were not all the same; I were beginning to tell 'em each one different, and now one of them had a name. She were folding her night clothes and I wondered at my being so afeared of her.

"See, you had nowt to be frightened of." Liza touched me on the shoulder.

"Susan's as dainty as they come. A high class lady's maid she was, a real lady herself."

"Then why's she here?"

"She's got the pox. There's many like her in here. Her 'usband brought it back from the South African War and ha' given it to her. There's nothing they can do for 'em."

"Are there no draughts, no medicines as will help?"

"Some of the doctors have tried giving 'em malaria, that's marsh fever as you know it, to see as if the fevers can drive the infection out, but for most of them it's too late anyway. But when they get too bad they move them onto the back wards, so do'an fret ye."

"What are the back wards?"

"Just like this one, but thems there are sicker and madder, scream and shout and fall down, or fight yer. They have rooms wi' the walls padded to put them in, call 'em the padds, and clothes and chairs that stop them using their hands to hurt the'selves… or others."

"Where are the back wards, Liza?"

"Have ye never seen 'em?"

"I've seen the old asylum from the road outside, but the walls are so high…"

"They call it the County Mental Hospital now, and the walls are high to keep us in. And the coping stones are smooth as if they're polished, and just as slippery, to stop us climbing over."

"But the gates are always open."

"Ay, but you and I can no more go through those gates than can that camel in the Holy Bible through the eye of a needle."

"I've seen the buildings over the wall. They look like the mills but not so big."

"Ay, for milling souls. On the one side is where they house the men and on the other the women. Two floors each building, red brick and all connected by corridors. And behind another row of buildings, just the same, but thems the back wards, behind the bell and the water tower, where they put them as frighten 'em. Where Susan 'll go if they think she's dangerous or they can't keep her clean and decent."

"Poor Susan."

"Now you be watching your step, or you'll be there yourself if you don' behave."

"Oh no, Liza, you're teasing me... aren't you? Have you been there?"

"Sure, and I've done my time there, but not again, they'll not make me go there again. Whatever they tell me. I am stronger now. I can fight them, I can fight them with their mind games. But away with your questions. I never met such a child for questions. Come, or we'll miss our breakfast."

II

I WATCHED AND I WAITED. I CLEANED WHEN
they said to, I ate what they gave me, and I walked round
and round and round the airing courts. Most of the ladies
stopped staring at me, and some even smiled. Liza told me their
names and sometimes I dared speak a few words to them. But
they were all so old, so much older than me. I thought of my
mother: she were old. I could tell when we shared a bed o' night:
she would curl round me to keep warm, and hold my hands,
and her fingers were fat and wouldn't bend proper, and when
she bent her knee into the bend of my knee I would feel it crack.

One day I told this to Liza as we walked.

"Liza, I think my mother was more poorly than these
ladies. She weren't strange like them, but she were always tired.
In the war she worked in one o' them munitions factories. She
came home all yellow, said she were a *canary girl*."

We were walking round the airing court as usual.

"I remember 'em. Worked hard, they did. We all did. I was
working as a housekeeper, but lots of the lasses in service went
to the factories to help the war effort."

"Me ma liked the work: said it were real work, like men's work. And it paid well. But it made her ill."

"I'll wager she never told them she had children. They mostly took the young 'uns, Mr Lloyd George's 'expendables'; made them 'cordite fodder', like the lads they sent to the Front. The old goat seduced them with wages like as they'd never seen before, and promises they'd be cared for."

"But she never stopped being yellow, after the war, and she were always coughing, Liza. Kept losing work 'cause of it."

"Sure you'll not find many as worked in them factories as are not ill now."

"She used to take me on the tram, after the war, down to where the Jewish ladies lived, 'cause they often wanted help on a Friday or a Saturday. And she'd leave me to wait outside while she went to 'door: but sometimes I'd creep up to the windows and look inside. And Liza, the houses were so warm and bright and cosy, and the clothes… and the children had such pretty little shoes. And when she got work there it were so good. She got good money and they gave her food as well, little pastries, like as I'd not seen before, and fruit, and fish as made a good pie. But they never took her on for long. But I don't see any Jewish ladies in here, Liza."

"No, child, surely they take care of their own."

"Oh, Liza, I do miss her. Why has she not spoken for me? After my brothers went to the Children's Village it were just the two of us. She took me everywhere with her. She hid me in her room when she got work in service. In her last place we were there for summat like two years and the cook found me out. She got me my work as a kitchen maid. They'll be needing me, they said I were a good worker."

"Mebbe."

"And I *were* a good worker, could do me mother's work as

well as mine when she were ill, and I were good at learning, though I never went to school."

"Did you never learn to read and write? Did your mother never read to thee?"

"She read me from the Bible, and she had a book of poems, but nowt else. I did start to go to school, but then me da was killed in the Somme battle and me ma started working in the factories."

"Well, they'll be giving you work in here soon enough."

"But I want to go home. 'Tis wrong I'm here. I see the doctor sometimes but they will na' let me speak to him. I've tried telling the Charge, but she willna' stop to listen, and the nurses say I must wait."

"Hush, child, you're warm and dry and fed well enough. Have patience." Then she pulled my arm through hers and patted my hand as she always did when we talked like this. And I put my t' other hand in the pocket of my apron to find the doll to hold.

Mostly Liza looked out for me, but there were days when she wouldna' speak to me and went off talking to herself. And she never would let me talk of my baby, my Peter, as I'd called him. Don't know why, just liked the name and I remembered it from me ma's Bible, and, as well, my mother used to say it meant "a rock", and rocks are strong. So my Peter would surely be strong; he must be safe and warm and fed now, but I feared for him, a deep, dark fear like I'd not felt before in all my life, though I'd been affrighted many a time. A fear that made me want to hide him away from anything as might hurt him.

None of t' other ladies were interested in me talking about my baby either. And I did so want to talk about him. My body was getting stronger, the griping pains in my belly were going, and the bleeding was stopping, but the needles would still prick in my chest, and the milk would still come when I thought on him.

Perhaps the nurses would understand. Now I was getting to know some of the ladies, I saw that the nurses were all different too. Some seemed cross all the time, but others seemed kindly, but they were all old. So old I dared not speak to them, except when I asked to see the doctor, and they always answered "no".

Then one morning one of the ladies spat in my porridge. Liza might say they were all ladies, but some of 'em were common as muck, and dirty an' all. "Witch!" she hissed at me. "Spying on me!" I stood up and screamed at her, "No, no, no, tha' shan't do that to me," but before I could hit her two of the nurses had hold of my arms, and were dragging me from the table. And I were hitting and kicking and trying to bite them, and screaming and screaming, "Leave me go, no, no, 'tis wrong. I shouldna' be here. They've stolen my baby. Get OFF of me. Le' me go. Le' me go."

And I kept fighting them and screaming as they bent my arm up my back till it hurt, and pulled and shoved me, with their feet and their hands and their elbows, along the corridor and back to the ward, where they lifted me by my arms and threw me on my bed. Then, as I sat up, one of them slapped me hard across the face, made me dizzy, and I fell back again so my head hit the bedhead, and I heard them saying they'd get the doctor and I'd be put where I couldn't hurt no-one if I didn't stop. And I remembered what Liza had said about the padds on the back wards, and I got frightened. So I quieted down, though my heart carried on beating so fast in my chest with the anger and the unfairness of it that I couldn't breathe. I didna' know I could be so angry, but now the anger had come up from deep, deep inside me, and filled me up and I wanted to hurt 'em all, like they'd hurt me. I hated them and I could've bitten and scratched them till they bled. But being angry had done me no better than keeping quiet. I was caught, like the rabbits Tommy and me had seen in gin traps, and there was no-one to help prise the jaws of the trap open to free me. The more I screamed and shouted the more they scorned me.

So when the rest of the ladies came back from breakfast, I just kept me head down, did the jobs I was given and said nowt more. And they said nowt to me, but I could see the nurses watching me, and my face was red raw from the slap they'd given me, and I could still taste blood from my lip, but I weren't going to let 'em see me cry again.

At midday we had our main meal, in the same great dining hall as we had our breakfast. The nurses took us there and watched over us as we ate. It were solid filling food, mainly stews, very, very often with rhubarb to fill us after. I were never left hungry. Most of the food, they said, came from the farm that were part o' the hospital, and I think they must have grown a great lot of rhubarb there.

I was shy of the nurses who stood over us as we ate, but I watched them, slyly, so they didn't see as I were watchin' 'em. Mostly they talked one to t' other and took little note of us. I think some of 'em had been working in the asylum just for ever, and they seemed to do the same things day in, day out, and we were a bother to them if we made them change. One day, in the airing court, I asked one of them if I might have a drink of water: the thirst that came after the birthing of my baby were less but still bad. They were there to care for us, I think, in a hard, distant sort of way, and we called them all by their Christian names, but there were little warmth in 'em, and when I asked they just said I must wait for water till we went back to the ward. They were kind of a part of the furniture of the place, same as we were, sort o' like the benches in the airing courts and the clock on the passage wall; and the faces that came and went scarce ever changed, though, once or twice, they were joined by a young woman or two whom I thought must be more my age, but they never stayed long enough for me to dare to mither 'em.

Then Molly arrived.

Molly was young, she had life, she made a noise, she made us laugh. She had sparkly eyes and thick corn-coloured hair, twisted into finger waves, and she was what me da would have called "comf'table".

She spoke to us, the patients, as she spoke to the other nurses, not hoity-toity but as if we were worth speaking to.

"I am one of the 'Surplus Women,'" she would say with her nose in the air, "and I'm proud of it! We may have lost our men in the trenches but we will be no-one's wizened widowed maiden aunts!" And the other nurses would half smile at her, as if they thought her as mad as the rest of us.

"'Tis better to have loved and lost," she would say, all sing-song, so she didn't seem to be in mourning. But ne'er had she time for our long slow-passing days and the idleness of the airing courts. I knew 'cause she'd wink at me, and yawn, and pretend to fall asleep. She'd make me giggle like as I was keeping her secret from t' other nurses.

Then, one afternoon, she came up to me as I was walking. "Mary, you're young and lively, don't you want to do something more than just walk round and round these paths all day?"

"What else could I do?"

"Have you never played hopscotch? No? Well come with me."

She took me to a corner of the airing court.

"Look, here's some tailor's chalk. We'll draw squares on the paving here like this. Now find a pebble from one of the flower beds and we'll use that as a marker. Now watch." And she lifted her skirts and hopped and jumped over the squares.

"Now it's your turn."

So I lifted my skirts and hopped into the squares, but I thought I would fall, mostly when I had to reach down and pick up the pebble, and then I'd put the wrong foot down, and I had to laugh. And I hopped and laughed and coughed till I could scarce breathe at all. Some of the ladies watched us but no-one tried to join in, and the other nurses turned their backs and "tutted".

"Molly, what if the Charge comes by? Will ye not be in trouble?"

"Never you mind. The exercise is good for us. This may not be very ladylike, but it's no worse than the Black Bottom they dance these days. I'd teach you that if we had the music and our skirts didn't so get in the way."

"One for sorrow,

"Two for mirth,

"Three for a funeral,

"Four for a birth.

"I'd love to dance, Molly."

"You'd be good at it if you didn't have two left feet. Hop on your *right* foot into that square."

"How do I remember which is my right foot?"

"Which hand do you favour? Then that's your right hand. Did no-one ever teach you right from left?"

"Yes, but I forget. Show me the Black Bottom."

"One day, not now, and not in these skirts. Now finish your turn: round at the top and hop back."

Then when I felt I had nowt more breath left in me I sat down on one of the benches, warmed through by all the hopping, face red and hot against the wind's chill, and Molly sat with me, panting like a man as had just chased a pig through a market. (I seen that once. It were very funny. It were not a very big pig, but the shop girls were squealing like they were the ones stuck!)

"So why are you here, Molly?"

"Ah well, that's a long story. After my husband, Donald, was killed on the Somme..." She struggled for the words through her gasps for breath, twisting her wedding ring on her finger. "He was shot leading his men over the top... very brave... they said... though I think they said that about every officer that died, didn't they? I helped in one of the hospitals that took the wounded when they were brought back home.

"Have you heard of the Somme battle in the Great War, Mary?"

"My father was killed on the Somme," I whispered. "I were six, but I remember. Me ma wouldn't stop crying."

"Ah so, then you have."

She was quiet again for a bit and I wiped my face with the corner of my apron and rubbed my legs where the wool of my skirt were itching them.

"After the war, I went back home to my family. I was meant to be married, indeed I *was* married, or had been, for all of a matter of days, before he went off to fight, but, as far as everyone was concerned, I'd had my chance. Anyway, we girls were fighting over the few men left. The casualties among the officer classes were much higher than among the men, you know, however they care to paint it."

That seemed an odd thing to say. They were dead or wounded whoever they were. But she carried on.

"It was all right to start with, parties, dances, even if it was three girls to a lad. But then my sister's children started to grow up. I could see myself turning into their ancient widowed aunt, all in black silk and smelling of lavender and moth balls, very good at japes, but not much use for anything else. So I decided I was going to find 'my vocation'. Do you know what that means, Mary? Find my calling in life. My mother didn't want me to come here, but the mental hospitals were the quickest way into nursing, so here I am!"

"Happen you like it, though, Molly?"

"Not much. I cried myself to sleep the first few nights I was here, stuck in a room in the nurses quarters, inside these walls, walking miles along the corridors to locked wards, no-one to talk to, no-one to laugh with, but I wasn't going to let them see me defeated. This is not my idea of nursing. There's little you can do for these women, no cure for their ailments. There's feeding and washing and dressing, keeping them safe. These old biddies that care for them are not nurses." She looked over at the women standing by the wall, scornin' them. "Some of the patients, like you, don't even need that."

"So, will you be for staying?"

"As long as I need to. It's a bit different on the back wards, where the patients are sicker, but even there there's little to be done for them. Sometimes it's just straightjackets to stop them harming themselves or others. I thought it would be different." I thought she looked sad.

"I'd seen the lads who came back with shell shock in the war, and I went to visit the Red Cross Hospital in Maghull, when they were trying to raise money for it. Dr Rivers talked to us about Freud and Jung and understanding the men's minds, and it sounded so exciting; mental illness that could be treated and even cured. But I don't see that kind of treatment, the 'talking treatments', here."

Then she sat up straight and took a deep breath. "But there *is* the infirmary wing, and there there's real illness and accidents that you can nurse, patients who get better, and even operations done sometimes (the doctors like doing those). Matron is a proper nurse and she wants us to get qualifications, in general nursing as well as mental nursing, and that's what I'm going to do."

"What's them qual-if-ic-ations, Molly?"

"Certificates, Mary, certificates that say you have learnt a lot.

"I shall bother her and the doctors to let me work in the infirmary, study my books at night and pass the exams. Then I can go and work in one of the big city hospitals, maybe even become a matron myself. Then my sister's children will say *look at Aunty Molly, she didn't need a man!*" And she bent over with laughter, between coughing and gasping for air, tucking her straying hair into their Kirby grips; though I thought her laughter were really sad, somehow, as if it were coming through a big black cloud.

"Oh, Mary, I shouldn't be telling you all this, child, but it won't mean anything to you. Now go and walk round or you'll get cold again."

"But why do we need men, Molly? I don't see as we need men, there've not been many men in my life. I remember me da, though. He used to lift me on his shoulders. We went to see him after he volunteered, when he were trainin' to be a soldier in the big park by Manchester. We got there on the train, me, me ma and me two brothers: Sam was only a baby. It were exciting, the steam engine pulling the carriages, and I liked the shiny wooden seats, and the leather handles on the window, and I got smuts in my hair when I put my head out the window. Then me ma smacked the backs o' me legs to make me come away from the window and sit down, but I was so excited I kept jumping up and down. I remember that better than me da. I just remember me ma huggin' him and crying when we left him. I s'pose I didn't know why he had to go away. If he didna' care for us, I wouldna' care for him."

"What did your mother do when he died?"

"She went into 'mournin', that's what she called it, but she were sad for she had no good black clothes to wear. But that weren't for long, then she got a job in a factory as what made the 'munitions', and she were reet happy again, 'cause she had money and friends and she were doing something important being a 'canary girl'. And that meant she could have Auntie Nell care for us. And Tommy and me, we 'bunked off' school and no-one chased us up, and the only man we ever saw was the charcoal burner in the wood."

"But did your mother not make you go to school?"

"Nah. But when the war ended she tried to settle us and make us a family again. Then me and Tommy started school again but we had to be in the 'infants', with the babies, as we couldna' read nor write, and I hated it. But all she had were a war widow's pension, and that weren't enough to keep and feed three children, so she took work and we moved around, and we didna' bother with school again, and she didna' care."

"I think she was ill-advised." Molly's voice were far away.

"It were hard for her."

"It was hard for all of us." Molly wasn't really listening to me now. I could see her looking at the other nurses and I thought she were more interested in them than me. I wanted to tell her about my baby, but off she went to find a mug of tea and join the other nurses, never mind what she'd said to me about them. I would ha' told her all about my Peter, if she'd ha' listened, but she weren't for hearing. She thought I were just a child, a child who knew nothing, who couldna' read nor write, an imbecile child who had a baby out of wedlock, a child of no importance to no-one...

But she made me think on me ma. Why *did* she never make us go to school? Why did she keep me when she sent the boys away? Why did she hide me so, away from the world, away from everything? Did she not want me to grow up? Why did we ne'er plan what was to be done wi' baby? Why did she leave me at the workhouse? Did she not truly care for me, for me as a real person? Or was I no more to her than this doll to me? Who am I really? And where is she now?

III

M Y FIRST WINTER IN THE HOSPITAL, THOUGH IT were still the asylum really, were cold and wet and windy. Oft-times we were kept from going out into the airing courts, and instead were sent to the big day room on the ground floor 'neath the ward. Here we could walk round the table for our "exercise", wearing a path across the wooden floor, or we could sit on the big chairs in front of the coal fire that were lit before we got there in the morning, or, they said, we could "play games". Some, those as knew how, could play draughts or backgammon or cards, but most didna' bother, they just walked or sat. There were a few books here as well, but I couldna' read them, and, sometimes, copies of the *Woman's Weekly* were brought in by visitors: we all jostled and fought over them, the nurses and us patients the same, to see the pictures in 'em mainly.

Then one morning the Charge, after her usual look at our work on the ward, said that today the mattresses on the beds should be checked. Those that were soiled were taken off the beds, four of us pulling at them to get them on t' floor, and then a two or three of us sat down to unpick the ticking covers of each one and remove the wiry horsehair and coir filling. I don't know why it should've been us as were chosen, but I didn't mind doing summat different for a change, and this was work I'd helped me ma with.

"Eurgh! Some of these covers should have been washed months ago!" Liza, though, didn't much like the work. "They smell, to be sure, worse than a dog's breath."

"It's real hard to pull the threads through, the cotton's reet heavy, it makes my fingers sore," I moaned, "but mebbe the seams are partin'. Look!"

"Just be glad it's only your fingers as are sore."

"Have I done enough? I can get my hand in to pull the stuffing out."

"No, unpick a bit further and then we can all pull the stuffing out together."

As the stuffing came out it filled the air with dust, sparkling in the little bit of sun coming through the windows, and settling on the sills and the bedheads, making more work for tomorrow's cleaning. We coughed and sneezed. I thought to myself, the nurses could've helped: they wouldn't have coughed and sneezed any more than they were anyway, and we might have been done quicker, but then Molly came over from where they were standing watching us.

"We need to tease it all out: it's become felted, all matted and flattened. Here, let me show you," and she pulled at the coarse wiry filling. "See, it fluffs up like eider down!" and she took a handful and tickled the back of my neck with it.

"It still feels scratchy to me. Look it's made me arms all red."

Molly took a handful and twisted it. "Look, now you have a bouquet. And if I pull this piece out so, you have a wig: the perfect bride!" And she took my hand and made me walk round the room.

Liza snorted, but I think it were a laugh she were hiding.

I felt foolish and my face were all hot, but Molly wouldna' leave go of my hand. Another lady, who'd never said a word to me afore, stood up and curtseyed to me. "Nay, she be no bride. She be the Queen o' the Fairies." And she laughed and laughed, and I just wanted to go away and hide meself.

Then Molly let go my hand and I slipped down onto the floor to me place with the mattress.

"Don't thee fret, they're not makin' fun o' thee, Mary. 'Tis just a game." Liza patted my hand.

"Tommy would've had fun with this," I whispered to Liza, but I could see others was listening. "He would have covered me in it till I cried out for him to stop. He did that with the piles of leaves that blew against the fence by the railway line. I wish he hadn't gone away, Liza."

"Never thee fret. Mebbe you'll see him again one day."

"No, I fear I willna'. We took him to the Children's Village, you know. Him and Sam. Me and me ma. It were two train rides and a good walk to the Village. Ma coughed and Sam cried, and when we got there I cried as well. It were just like a proper village, like you see in pictures (Auntie Nell had a picture. It were called 'The Village Green', she said, been gi'en her by someone as couldna' pay her for her carin' for their children), with houses with gardens wi' flowers at t' front and white-painted fences, and gates, all set round a bit o' green grass and trees, where children were playin'. We had to go to the first house, which weren't a house at all, it were like a police station, with a counter and desks and people writing in ledgers." I had stopped whispering and I could see more ladies were listening.

One of them bent forward. "I remember a village like that, near London, where I came from. It were Dr Barnardo's. There were girls as well as boys, but they were kept in different places. What happened to your brothers?"

"Me ma said she'd brought her boys because she couldn't look after them no more, and a man came and took us into one of the rooms. He asked the boys' names and how old they were, and what had happened to their father. Then he said, "Right, boys, we'll find someone to take you to your house. Say goodbye to your mother, and no crying, boys here don't cry." And a lady came and took them away, even though she had to pull Sam's fingers off my mother's skirt, he held on so tight."

"But they would have been happy there, surely?" Molly frowned. "I've heard of these homes too: they are said to give wonderful new opportunities to poor children."

"I don't know. We weren't allowed to see where they'd be. They said that was too 'unsettling' for em. And they said, no visiting for the first month, as visiting was 'unsettling' as well. So we had to go home, and never did see where they were taken.

"We did go visit them, twice. But it were a long way, and Sam cried and wanted to come home with us, and me ma cried, and Tommy tried to be all grown up and said he was going to be a soldier and ran off with his friends. And then one day me ma got a letter saying that Sam and Tommy had been 'emigrated' to Canada. There was nowt she could do. She tried, of course: we went back to the Village, but she couldn't get them back, and the Children's Village promised her they would have a better life in a new country. There would be fresh air and jobs for them and they would be well cared for. So she just gave herself up to never seein' 'em again."

"So you don't know where they are now?"

"No, and I do wish I could see them again."

"But they will have a good life in the colonies, new young countries with new young people: what an adventure for them."

"But they were just children. I came from Ireland." Liza's voice were hard, but she spoke slow and quiet, "with a 'usband and such hope for the new country, but I was sore lonely. Children need their families."

"Not if their families can't support them."

"But with just a little help me ma could have looked after them."

"But she couldn't, could she? Society cannot support every individual who fails to make their way, every bastard child that gets born, or every widowed mother's sons. Better they benefit from schemes like that. Ah, enough!" Molly turned back to the mattress covers. "Now, away with this one for washing, and here's a new cover to fill."

And we set to, repacking the teased-out filling into the fresh ticking. After that the seams had to be stitched together again. I helped, but the skin on my fingers was soft, and it were difficult to force the blunt needles through the thick cotton.

"Sure, and those are nifty stitches you're sewing, Mary. Would you care to join us in the parlour of an afternoon?" I knew Liza was teasing me but I didna' like her voice: it were all sing-song with hard edges. "We shall take tea and 'broider her ladyship's doilies. Then we can talk o' how we'll rid this country of its undeserving."

I smiled, but Molly was frowning and Liza looked cross, even though she were laughing. "I would like to do some work, though," I said. "I've not sewn before, but I could learn."

But no-one was listening to me, and now Molly was sharp. "They should be grateful of the opportunities."

"Ah, yes, Mrs High and Mighty Charity Lady, come to make all our lives better. Surely you've never missed an 'opportunity'!"

"Don't you dare speak to me like that, madam. I know you're clever, Liza, and I know you have the ear of some as should know better. And don't think I don't see you, talking union talk with the girls that come in here to work, but you'll not change the world, you'll not get the idle off the streets with your 'welfare', you'll not get better wages by bankrupting the men who know how to run the country and make its wealth..."

"Ha, organised greed. 'Twill only be defeated by organised labour."

Molly walked away and Liza turned to me again. Her hands were shaking. She took a deep breath and sat up very straight, then, "Jesus, Mary, there's plenty of sewing to do, but they're looking for seamstresses and tailors to make these horrid skirts for us and the uniforms for the nurses. But there's the laundry as well you could work in. You'll have to wait till you've seen the doctor again."

I sighed; surely the doctor would let me go and I wouldna' need the work.

But then I had another thought. Molly had said Liza was clever. "Liza, you can read, can't you? Happen you can teach me? I never went to school long enough to learn. And then I can show my Peter when he grows."

"My child, I shall teach you what you want. And then, one day, you can write the story of the lost women, who spent their days mending mattresses and talking to the moon."

And Liza did what she promised. Somewhere she found a slate and a piece of chalk, and in the mornings in the airing courts or, better still, in the day room, she taught me the alphabet, and then how to put the letters together to make words. I loved it. I just loved it, it were such fun. I loved making the curls and the loops with the chalk, and it were such a joy when I first wrote my own name. "But I still can't make no sense of the words in the *Woman's Weekly*, Liza."

"You will, one day." Then Liza took a book from her apron. It were bound in a red cloth cover with gold writing and black curls on it, and it was as big as a man's hand and as thick as my thumb.

"This is my treasure, Mary. It was given me and I take it everywhere. You can see it's surely been well read. It says here, *Mrs Beeton's All about Cookery, New Edition 1909*. And here inside are advertisements, like kind of recommendations for things to buy, look, here's one for refined beef suet. It tells you to make rice pudding with shredded suet – for feeding delicate children, poor things." She followed the writing with her finger. "And if you look further inside, indeed, there are recipes, that's how to make foods like pies 'n puddings; and there's advice for the housewife as well. One day I shall be running a little guesthouse, I shall, that is my dream, and this will be my Bible. But for now you may use it to learn to read. And we shall start at the beginning, with the recipes starting with A. Look, here, alma pudding."

Then, day by day, I began to work with Liza on the print on *Mrs Beeton's* pages. I liked the recipes as much as I liked readin' 'em, and I would try to think how I would make them, remembering what I'd learnt when I worked as a kitchen maid. Then Molly teased me, "And who's the little bookworm then?" and I boasted of my new reading skills to the ladies I shared my life with, who watched me and who talked to themselves. And I forgot to be frightened of them, and I learnt from Liza how to help them, and who to keep away from, and how to close my eyes and my ears to the sights and sounds as they talked in their sleep, or wandered the ward at night, or worse. Then, as Liza had said, Susan left to go to one of the back wards, "Where the doors are locked all the time, missy," one of the nurses warned, "and there's no hope of you ever leaving, and where they shut you in with the worst and wait to see how long you go before you cry to be let out!"

"Poor Susan," I said to Liza. "What will she do?"

"Happen she'll die there, one day, and may the Good Lord hold her safe in the palm o' His hand till then, there's nowt you nor I can do for her now."

IV

THE BEDS WERE ALWAYS FULL OF A NIGHT. As Liza's "ladies" like Susan left, their places were filled by others.

One night on beds close to mine there were two new women, young like me. They were both beautiful, leastways I thought them beautiful, but then I were just used to the old biddies I saw on the ward every day. They didna' speak to me and I wouldna' dare speak to them, though I were curious, so I just watched them. One of 'em was tall and thin, with her hair all red curls over her shoulders and down her back. She knelt on her bed and rocked herself to and fro, folding the corner of the blanket over and over to make perfect straight creases then smoothing them out again. If anyone came near her she screamed and screamed, and she wouldna' take her clothes off as bidden. I think she must have stayed like that all night as she were still kneeling there when I woke the next morning.

T' other was smaller, with thick black hair and skin as pale as the milk when you've skimmed the cream off it. She were lying curled up on the bed with her face covered. And when they told her to get in the bed she took off her outdoor clothes (they were soft silks and perfectly stitched white cottons, and I thought *that's the last you've seen of those, missy*) and she slipped into the bed without a word. But she didna' sleep and most of the night, whenever I woke, she were walking up and down, up and down, till daybreak, when she got back into her bed and had to be shaken awake by the nurses when the day bell rang. They called her Ruth, and she did as they bade her and dressed in the skirts and aprons we all had, and I saw her eyes were dark as well and sunken into dark hollows in her cheeks.

But the red-haired lass didna' move, though they gave her her new clothes and shouted at her, "Agnes, get dressed!" She just shrieked again, as soon as they came close to her. Then one of the nurses caught hold of her arm, and now it were the nurse as were screaming as she'd bitten her hand. And the nurse hit her hard across her face and her head hit the bedstead, but she didn't cry, she just screamed even more, and Liza appeared from nowhere and shouted at the nurse, "Sure, can ye not see she's frightened out of her wits? Jesus, Mary and Joseph, if you box her ears like that, I'll box yours, you mark my words. Now leave her to me."

And Liza sat down on the bed a little away from where the poor girl was knelt and started to talk to her. "Now, Aggie, there's no need to be afeared, the ladies here will no harm thee. Tha's Mary and I be Liza, Leeeeeza, mind, not Lie-za, and not Elizabeth, nor anything else, and we're in the County Mental Hospital, and we'll go for our breakfast, but we all must be dressed first..." and she kept on talking and handing the clothes to Aggie, who shrank away from her but stopped screaming and became calmer. Then she led her, without touching her, so she could wash, and Aggie wouldn't look at her but she did as she should, and when she was ready followed Liza as we all went to breakfast.

Then at breakfast Aggie rearranged her porridge and her bread till it was to her liking, but then she ate it all, every scrap, though she still would not look at anyone nor let anyone touch her, and she still did not speak at all. And everyone watched her, so no-one except me saw that Ruth stirred her porridge round and round her bowl but did not eat a mouthful.

But Liza cared. "Come, Mary, we have two little strays here who need our help. Bring Ruth and show her the way, and we will make them comfortable."

And all morning Aggie followed Liza around and I got cross with her as Liza'd never cossetted me like that. "She is just like your little lapdog, Liza!"

"Be patient, child. I've seen 'em like this before. You must help me. She will settle when she knows the routine. But she is in danger. They will have no time for her if she screams all the time, and she doesna' deserve to be on the back wards. We must protect her. And that one, Ruth, that one will just get forgotten if thee and me don't look out for her."

So I stamped my feet as I did my work on the ward to show I was cross, but at the same time I was a little bit pleased that Liza wanted me to help her, and when we went out to the airing courts I took Ruth's arm to guide her, and I walked with Liza as she watched over Aggie. I couldn't figure out how much Aggie understood. She still didn't speak at all and yet she seemed to understand Liza, or was it just that she copied everything Liza did?

I looked for Molly. Perhaps she could explain. But she wasn't there; I would have to wait to ask her my questions.

In the meantime I tried to talk to Ruth. Though she would speak when spoken to, she said very little. I thought I would ask her how she were feeling.

"Tired," she said, "always tired, and no use to anyone. I can't understand why I'm alive."

"Is that 'cause you're here? I felt a bit like that sometimes when I came."

"No, that's *why* I'm here. I came voluntarily. The doctors say I have melancholia. They told my husband they might be able to make me better in here."

"Did they say you were ill, then? Why did you get ill?"

"I don't know, Mary. How can I answer your questions? I had a baby, it was after that."

"I had a baby too. They *made* me come here."

"Don't ask me any more, Mary. I can't help you. I don't want to talk to anyone about it."

"But did you have a boy or a girl? I need to know. I don't know where my little boy is and I miss him so."

"A boy, but I couldn't care for him. He didn't love me and I didn't love him. Or perhaps I did love him. Too much. I don't know. Please don't ask me anything more."

"So where is he?"

"Mary…" and she turned away from me and sat down on one of the benches (we were in the airing courts), and put her head in her hands. Liza came up.

"Don't worry at the poor lass, Mary. She'll tell you more in time, I dare say."

"But how can she have left her baby? All I want in all the world is to find my Peter again. 'Tis not fair."

"Did I not say to thee, you'll see the Devil's work all round you in here. She needs your help, not your anger. And babes, more 'n all, they're the Devil's work."

"I *shall* not speak to her then, if that's what tha' wants," and I walked away to mind my own thoughts and left them. I didna' care if they didn't want me. And I weren't going to mind that Aggie either, Liza's little pet. She were walking round the airing court, seeming counting her steps and turning reg'lar after so many. She had her hands over her ears but she were smiling, though to herself, not to anyone I could see.

So I bided my time till I could speak to Molly.

I caught her one morning while we were making our beds.

"Tell me about Ruth and Aggie, Molly. Ruth says she had a baby," I whispered.

"That she did, and then she developed melancholia and couldn't take care of it."

"So what's happened to it?"

"Being cared for by her sister, I believe."

"Does she no love it?"

"I expect she does, but she talked of killing it, and herself, and she couldn't feed it. It was all they could do to get her to dress herself, and her husband couldn't afford someone to care for her as well as for the baby. So he had to let her come in here."

"But surely she could have tried. I…"

"Mary, she's sick. She doesn't want to feel like this."

"But…"

"Help her, Mary, we must try to make her strong again, but no-one knows what's wrong with Aggie. Could be mania, or dementia praecox, so say the doctors."

"Them long words mean nowt to me, Molly. Can't hardly say 'em, let alone know 'em."

"All I know is she has these attacks. You've seen her screaming. She lived with her family till they could cope no more. And then she started forcing herself on men who came to the house. They had to keep her locked up. It's a sad story for I think they loved her. But the doctors tried calming her with bromide and it only made her worse."

"She doesn't speak, Molly."

"No, but she may *understand* you so you should try to speak to her."

"She follows Liza everywhere."

"She seems to learn by watching, and Liza is very patient with her."

"Ay, like as she were something special."

"Well, maybe she is. Look at her just now: she's making patterns of the shadows of her fingers on the wall. I don't know what they are, but they almost seem to be dancing."

"Huh, be better use helping fold these sheets."

V

I T FELT LIKE SPRING HAD COME THAT DAY THEY
took me to see the doctor again. I had walked round
and round the airing courts, day in and day out through
the cold, wet and windy days of winter. Could've walked the
London Road in all that time. But that morning the sun was
shining again. It didn't seem to make much difference to Aggie,
pacing, pacing, half a turn, pacing, pacing, half a turn, and
always in the same direction. But the sun! It were warm on my
face and it shone through Aggie's hair like the beams through
the cobwebs as they came through the windows of a morning;
like the halos round the heads of the saints in the pictures in
me ma's Bible. She were beautiful, Aggie, she would have liked
those pictures. She was real taken with circles and anything
that turned in circles. There were a great clock, like I'd only
ever seen before in the railway station the time we'd travelled
to see my father. It were on the wall along the corridor on our
path out to the airing courts, and every day Aggie stopped in
front of it. If I took her arm to pull her away from it she would
scream and scream and put her hands over her ears, so we all

knew to leave her be. When she were ready and she'd had her fill of watching the hands move she'd follow the rest of us.

"Aggie, come sit with us."

She never looked at me when I called. She might as well never have heard. But she came and sat beside me on one of the benches and started playing with my hair. She followed me everywhere now instead of Liza, and I weren't jealous of her no more. Indeed, I counted her my friend.

"Why do 'e care to touch my hair, Aggie, when you won't let no-one touch you? You willna' tell me? Ah, well, feel that sun on your face."

I lifted my face to the sun, but Aggie would not look, and Ruth was in a dream as if she were a long, long way away. Even Liza's forehead was creased peevishly. "It'll do none of us any good, heating our blood, making false promises, giving us hope!"

"But, Liza, at least it's warm."

"So, my dear, is hellfire."

I felt cold inside me, deep in my stomach, when Liza was grumpy like this. I went to take her hand, but she put it under her apron, and her eyes looked hard yonder past me.

"Liza, are you sad?"

"Now what would be the point of that?"

"Then art' angry with me?"

"No, not with thee, though b' Jesus I shall be if you carry on. Now, get away with you, I shall sit here for a wee while. You must walk again. Take them with thee," and she turned away.

I stood and turned my face to the sun again, but its warmth had gone. I wanted me ma, I wanted my baby.

Then one of the nurses came up to me. "The doctor's waiting to see you, Mary, come with me."

Down the wide corridors we went. I wanted to skip along them. I'd waited so long for this. I'd asked and asked to see the doctor. This was my chance to get out of here and find me ma and my baby. We came to the little room with the benches and the great door, and then, when I was called into the doctor's room, to the great desk behind it. It were a different doctor this time. I think he were younger. This time he looked at me with fine blue eyes that seemed almost to smile at me, and yet… not. He looked in my eyes for what seemed a good time, and I tried to look straight back at him, but I couldna', though I were smiling with hope inside me. Then he took my hands and turned them over. "How are you, Pearson?"

"I am well, sir, can I go home?"

He turned to the nurse, letting go my hands, and without waiting she reached for me, led me to the side of the room and undressed me. All the same again! I stood on the rattling step of the weighing machine, till she prodded me across the room. The doctor looked as if he were thinking, then he smiled. He looked at my skin and parted my hair, my thin, straight hair, the colour of dusty sand, that had thickened for the baby and was now falling out in handfuls. He listened to my chest, and put his hand upon my stomach. Then he turned me around and ran a finger down from my neck to the bottom of my back, such as made me shiver. Then he let his hand rest on my bum, just soft and gentle, just for a wee while, but it made my face go all red and hot.

He didna' seem to notice. "She has gained weight," he said to the nurse as he wrote in the ledger in front of him on the desk. "She is less pale. She has some alopecia. The hair often thins after childbirth; but her body appears to be responding to the feeding regime here, and she has no lice.

"You may dress her."

"Why am I here, sir? Mayn't I go home? Where is my baby?"

"Pearson – Mary – your baby will have gone to a wet nurse, and most likely a man and wife will be found who will adopt it."

"But I can care for him, my mother will help."

"Where is your mother, Mary?"

"I don't know, sir."

"Mary, did you know you were with child? Did your mother know?"

"Yes, sir, she said I weren't to tell no-one or we'd both lose our positions."

"Mary, can you tell me how you came to be with child?"

Something seemed to press on my heart and I was breathing faster and faster. I was dizzy. I wanted to cry.

"No, sir."

"Breathe slowly and deeply, Mary; do you understand what I asked?"

"Yes, sir."

"Then tell me."

"I cannot, sir."

With a sigh he turned back to the desk. "Mary, you cannot look after yourself; how could you possibly care for a baby? Society sees fit to protect sinners such as yourself, from yourselves and from your base urges, and to lead you, and those that you would lead, away from temptation. Do you understand? They call you and your like 'the morally defective'. Many would say it's society's duty to prevent you producing more defectives. You slipped through the net once, but you may be sure your baby will have a good Christian upbringing and be fitted for a clean and moral life, and hopefully his inheritance will have been purged of your bad blood." To the nurse, "We will see her again in another half year."

My hands were shaking, and I could see nothing for me tears. What did he mean? My baby would ha' grown up kind and good and funny like Tommy. Well, p'raps a bit naughty but not *bad*. I were not *bad*.

I was dressed again and the nurse took my shoulders and pushed me out the door, from where someone else took me back down the corridors to the ward. There I found my doll once more and slipped again onto the floor behind the bedstead. Again I felt the needles in my chest, but now the milk didn't come, but the tears wouldna' stop. And that was how I was when Liza came looking for me.

"Liza, how could I answer? How could I tell 'em it were the house, the house where me ma and I were working? She said I were to tell no-one: we would lose our positions, and this had been a good 'un. She'd worked there since I were thirteen, and the cook had found me out, hidin' in me ma's room, and got me a place as kitchen maid." I were crying so hard I could hardly get the words out.

"Hush." Liza took the corner of her apron and wiped my face. She was sat beside me on the floor. It weren't till after that I wondered how she'd got there: they'd locked me in when they left me. But then Liza did things others couldna'.

"Would have done thee no good to have told 'em, mark my words," she said.

"We had a room at the top, under the eaves, Mother and me, that you got to up the back stairs, Liza," I sobbed. "There were a boy, the 'young sir' we called him. He were away at some posh school most of the time, used to see him when he came home in his top hat 'n all. When he came back for Christmas he brought a friend with him."

"You don't need to tell me, Mary. Holy Mother, how often have I heard this story. Sure, Adam was the first sinner, but women have been paying ever since."

"They were not much in the house, Liza, the young sir and his friend, and never in the kitchen, but they were handsome boys, they were, always laughin' and playing games, and sometimes they came up the back stairs and they'd find me on my own."

"So what did they do to you, my child? Though it takes little imagining."

"At first they just wanted me to take my clothes off, just to see, they said. I was too frightened to say no. But they didn't hurt me. Then they wanted to touch, and stroke my breasts and put their fingers between my legs, and I was frightened, but it felt good as well, and wet and warm, and I knew it must be sinful. Oh, Liza, why did I let them?"

"The Good Lord knows. Tha were just a child thasel'."

"And then the friend went home, Liza, 'n James came on his own, and he locked the door and told me lie on the bed. He held me down by my shoulders, and knelt over me, and then he pushed himself into me, and it hurt, and yet it didn't hurt, and I didna dare make a noise. And quickly it was over, and I cried and cried, but quietly, and there was blood, and I knew I were a sinner, but he were laughing and panting like a little dog, and I felt dirty and angry, but, Liza, it were worse: at the same time I wanted to hold him, and I wanted him to hold me, and… how could I tell 'em? It were my fault.

"He said that he were sorry, and he did look sorry, and a bit afeared, but that I mustn't tell. And I didn't, but he came back again. And sometimes he kissed me, wet, soggy kisses with his tongue in my mouth. And once he said he thought I was beautiful. And Liza, I didna' stop him. And then he went back to school. And I started to get fat, and mother noticed, so I had to tell. But she made me promise as well, never ever to tell anyone else. So how could I tell the doctor?"

"You're still no more 'n a child yourself. It were wrong of thee, but he should have had to pay. Now look at ye. How are you going to grow up in a place like this? And are you still clutching that doll? His joints are rusting now and, for sure, his face has been washed away by your tears. Now what possessed them to treat you like a child when you were a mother?" She looked away, far into the distance, as if she were somewhere else. "Ah me, they said I couldna' be a mother, and I believed them, but that were a long time ago and I was not strong then." She looked at me again and her voice grew louder again. "I am strong now. And you must be strong, and your baby will live and grow into a man."

"What do you say, Liza?"

"Never thee mind. Now give me the doll and go wash your face," so I gave her the doll, and I felt better for telling her what I'd done. But I felt the shame again.

"But Liza, my baby was beautiful. Mebbe it were wrong, but I loved him, I loved him so much."

"He were the Devil's gift, but that were not his fault, poor child. But you must forget him. He is gone, but surely he is safe.

"Come now, look at that, Mary, see how the sun's shinin' still, and it's warming the flowers on the table there."

That made me smile. It were no time since Liza were grumpy with me for sayin' the sun were warming. Now she were telling me of its warmth to cheer me. But I were still sad. My chance to see the doctor, to tell him why I should be home, to get to see me ma and my baby, had been wasted. Liza was right. I needed to be stronger, and cleverer.

"I know them flowers, Liza. They're daffodils. They used to grow by the railway line where me 'n Tommy went: I think someone had mebbe planted them once to cheer the coalmen up! The charcoal burner called them Lent lilies, and he said they bloomed in the garden of Geth-sem-ane before Christ's Last Supper. They mean there to be great sorrow but hope as well."

"Well, Jesus, Mary and Joseph, there's a story for you, child. Now let's go down to the airing courts, the nurse is waiting to take us. We'll have no more talk of babies."

VI

I T WERE THAT DAY THAT I SAW THE DOCTOR THAT turned me: if I were to learn to read and write I might find a way out of this place and back to my baby. If I could read books I might understand how it could happen that you could be locked up for having a baby. And if I could talk proper I might be able to argue with 'em. So I sat with Liza in the day room, day in, day out, staring at the letters in *Mrs Beeton*, copying them onto the slate and trying to make sense of them. I liked the recipes as well, and, as I copied the letters, I'd learn 'em so I could tell them to myself when I was in bed or walking in the airing courts, and I'd got nothing better to think of.

Sometimes then I'd tell them to one of the other ladies, or to Aggie, or Liza. Liza would listen but no-one else would, though Aggie would say them back to me, all sing-song, sometimes days after, just as if she knew what they were.

"Liza, I like the recipes in your book; have you cooked them all?" I asked one day as we sat in the day room.

"Nay, bless you. When would've I had time for fancy cooking?"

"'Cause I think I could do some of 'em better. There were things I learnt when I were a kitchen maid, and some things me ma told me, or the charcoal burner, when me 'n Tommy found him in the woods. And mebbe I might make 'em pretty, like as the little pastries the Jewish ladies made."

"My, what a dreamer y' are. Sure 'n you need to get your hands dirty again with some proper work."

"Well, they're dusty enough from the chalk, see." And I wiped my fingers down the side of her skirt, making white trails like a dusty snail. I thought she might slap me but she laughed.

"Be gone with thee, child. I'll have nowt to do with y' messin'. Now get on with writing or I'll leave ye."

So I leant over my slate again and started copying "Queen of Puddings".

Molly came by and sat beside me and watched me for a while. "One of the visitors has given me some butcher's block paper, Mary. Here, try writing on this," and she handed me a folded sheet of thick buff paper and a lead pencil. The pencil felt strange in my fingers after the chalk, but I spread the paper out and tried writing my name.

"Look, Molly, I can make the loops and curls of my name so pretty with the pencil, and… a flower. Look, just like a daisy."

Aggie came to see. She took the pencil from me and started to draw circles, lots and lots of circles, like bubbles. She held the pencil just so, as if she'd been taught to write proper; and the bubbles were truly round, not just scribble. But then she dropped the pencil and walked away.

"She were taken with the bubbles when we bathed, Molly, though she couldna' get many from t' 'ard soap they ha' gi'en us. But the paper's good. Canst find us more?"

"I have plenty, Mary. I'll make it into smaller sheets for you, and you can write your recipes on them. And we'll find a place here in the day room where you can keep them, and some pencils too. You're doing well with your writing, and you'll be reading other books soon. Well done."

"And Aggie can draw her bubbles as well, if she wants."

"Jesus, Mary and Joseph, I'll be runnin' a school here soon," Liza grumbled, but I think she was quite proud of us really. Sometimes she were right down, but other days she made us feel we could all be more than just sick, helpless women. Like when we bathed.

We bathed once a week, ten of us at a time, each in a big iron bath with water the nurses tested for heat. We had to line up after we'd taken all our clothes off, so as they could look us over for cuts and bruises, or scabs and lice. I was shy and I felt shamed, even though I was used to the bath houses me ma took me.

But Liza made us lift our heads. "We shall surely show them we are ladies of breeding. We shall stand straight and proud as we walk to the baths, and we shall sing whilst we wash." But all we knew were hymns, so we started off, just quiet to start with, "Dear Lord and Father of mankind, forgive our foolish ways..." then louder, until the sound echoed off the shiny green tiles on the walls and I thought they'd hear us in the road outside the asylum walls.

Liza knew all the words and kept us going. And so did Aggie. Aggie could sing every hymn we tried, and as well as the words she knew all the tunes perfectly. When we sang "Dear Lord and Father," the rest of us would fall quiet as we forgot the words, (that one were not a hymn many of us had learnt as children) but Aggie's sweet high voice would carry on right up to the last "Still small voice of calm". She sang like I thought only an angel could sing, and it made us all feel very clean and pure, till Liza made us laugh again. "Sure, ladies, we sing like pink piglets released from purgatory!" But it felt like I'd said to the nurses, "This is me, and even if you have charge of me I'm as good as thee." And I think t' others felt the same. And mebbe the nurses saw us as real women for a while and not just mad or bad or sick.

But I was sad when I saw Ruth. I couldn't forgive her for leaving her baby, but when I saw her in the bath I felt sick at the scabs on her arms where she'd picked the skin, and at how thin she were. They tried to make her eat, but she wouldna'. They took her away to weigh her every week, and they fed her bread and Marmite ('cause the nurses told us one of the doctors had said they'd tried feeding Marmite to starving people in India, wherever that was, whose blood was thin like Ruth's). Then they tried giving her cod liver oil and malt as well. But it didn't do no good. I felt mebbe I should tell her. "Ruth, canst tha not eat, for the sake of t' baby?"

"The food sticks in my throat. I cannot stomach it."

"But for your baby?"

"Mary, every Sunday my husband brings him in to see me. We sit in the dining hall and I hold him, and I feel nothing. I just want to die. He is better off without me."

"But can ye not try to feel better for him?"

"If I could do that, would I be here? You don't understand. How could you: your life is so uncomplicated."

"If tha's saying I'm simple, well mebbe I am, but, Ruth, tha' walks at night, back 'n forth, can tha not sleep? If tha' slept tha' might save strength for t' baby."

"I am tired but I cannot sleep, Mary."

"Aggie could sing to you."

"Mary, I am not a child to be sung lullabies to. Neither do I care for your pestering."

"Then I cannot help thee."

And I walked away from her. I was trying to help. Deep in my stomach I felt I should care about her, but I found it so hard that she should see her baby every week and I knew nowt of mine. I was a mother too. She might think me a simpleton, but I was still sad for my baby, and for hers.

VII

THE NIGHTS WERE NEVER-ENDING THROUGH the long days of summer. The sun still shone through the windows when we went to bed, and after the key had been turned, scraping and jangling, in the lock on the ward door. Some of the ladies were used to it and they went straight to sleep, but I couldna'. I'd lie in my bed and look up at the ceiling, and I'd try saying my recipes out loud, just whispering, mind. And I'd pretend I were writing on the sheets with my finger. And sometimes I'd try out some numbers. Molly was teaching me arithmetic: she said I needed to be able to add and subtract and multiply if I were to understand the weights and measures in my recipes. Some of the tiles under the windows had bumps on them like teeth, so I'd count the number on each tile, then I'd count the number of tiles and try to work out how many teeth there were on the whole wall. Molly was teaching me times tables but mostly I still did things on my fingers. There were seven teeth to each tile and four tiles under each window, but then twenty-eights were too many to work out any further just on my fingers.

Sometimes I'd watch Ruth when she got out of bed and walked up and down the middle of the room, and sometimes just watching her would send me to sleep.

Then from time to time a nurse would come by and look in on us, and the grating of the key in the lock would wake me again.

One night I were still awake when it went dark. I could hear Aggie tossin' and turnin' in the next bed. She still said nowt to us though she would copy what *we* said, and sometimes she'd even copy our voices, so good you couldn't tell who'd spoken. Some of the ladies thought she were scornin' them, but she didn't mean harm by it, and she weren't laughing at them. I still thought she were beautiful. Her hands and her hair were so soft. And her skin looked like it were shining, I think because it were so pale. Not pale ill like Ruth's, but pale and silken, like the petals of a white dog rose in the hedge.

I heard her get out of bed, the slap of her bare feet on the floor. She came to the side of my bed and started to climb in. It was difficult to make room for her: my body had made me a dip in the middle of the mattress just big enough for me, so Aggie was tipping onto me from the side. She pulled my chemise up and stroked my breasts and squeezed them, then she pulled her own chemise up and I felt her leg moving over the tops of mine, and she was moving against me, her fanny rubbin' on the bone of my hip. I didna move. What should I do? But, oh, it felt so good, the warmth of her skin on mine, the soft roundness of her belly, even the hard dig of her elbows.

Then she sighed, and went all soft and sleepy beside me. I wanted to shift so she could move into the dip beside me, but I couldna. And anyway, she were soon away, back to her own bed as quick as she came.

And that was how it happened. My beautiful Aggie coming to my bed in the dark, not speaking, not staying, but

I learnt to make it good for me as well as her. And it changed nowt in the day.

But we were not the only ones as shared a bed o' night. We all knew about when in the night the nurses would come to check on us and tried to be in our own beds then, but even if we weren't, so long as they could head count us they didn't mostly care; only if they were after you for something else would they take you before the Charge the next day and she'd call you "depraved", whatever that meant, and mebbe you'd be punished, have to stay on the ward, or sweep the corridors or summat, instead of going to the airing courts. But most of the ladies did it for comfort and warmth as much as anything. It were sometimes very lonely in that big room with the ceiling so high above us, even if there were so many beds with so many souls in them.

Then on Sundays we trailed off to church, so God could get a good look at us and we could pray, as the nurses said, for our "deliverance" from whatever had got us into this place. We were led, two by two like schoolchildren, by the nurses, who made sure we were kept a good distance from the men patients, who sat in the pews on the other side of the aisle. It were a chapel really. Not that big, but of course it only had to make room for those of us in the front wards none of the "difficult" patients from the back wards ever came. But it were a proper chapel, with coloured glass windows the sun shone through, and a big altar, and an organ for playing the hymns. I liked the walk to the services. We were still inside the hospital walls, but the paths took us past the cricket ground and some of the vegetable plots, and I could see where all that rhubarb came from.

The nurses came to church, of course, and some of the doctors. It was there I first saw the Superintendent, though he didn't come often. He were tall and walked with a stoop, peeking through his thick glass spectacles, and always looking worried. They said he took to his bed of a Sunday with blinding headaches, so he would send his wife and children to church in his stead. I thought they were very brave: they were the only people there from "outside". His wife were so pretty. She had her hair cut in the new style "bob" like we'd seen in the *Woman's Weekly*, and she wore suits with skirts that came only just below her knees: we'd talk about her clothes for days after. Five children she had, three boys and two girls, and sometimes they'd stop on their way out to speak to a nurse, or a patient. Some of the patients had been here for years and years, like many of the nurses, so I suppose they got to recognise them, and we were all very respectful.

I'd been to church when I were younger, of course, but not much: enough to like the Bible stories I'd heard, and to believe in a God who'd made everything in seven days, and then given his Son to save us from Hell. And when we were little, mother had read us from the Bible she kept by her bed, and I loved the sounds of the words, and the patterns they left in my head when she stopped speaking. And I loved the hymns as well, and, though I didn't go to school much and I couldna' read them, they stayed like poems in my mind, to be said out loud when Tommy and I were on our own, sometimes making up new words for them when we couldna' remember the right ones. So I found the church services very safe and comforting, and I would happily join in the singing.

One of the Charges had got some of the patients together to make a choir. They were good enough to be allowed sometimes to sing in the village church "outside"; the gossip was that the Charge was so proud of his work he wanted to take them even further away to show 'em off. Of course, it wasn't long before one of our nurses told him about Aggie, and her singing at bath times.

I were sitting next to her when he came over. I always sat next to her in church to make sure she were not unhappy or frightened. Liza was never there. The Catholics had their services in the dining hall, for there weren't so many of 'em. He spoke straight to her.

"I hear you have a good ear for a tune and you know all the words to the hymns, my girl."

She wouldna' look at him, so I said, "I think she would sing in your choir if you wanted, but I'd have to sit with her till she got used to it."

So I did, and she were happy with that. So long as she didn't have to do owt different she sang when a tune was played, whether others sang with her or not. And her voice was so beautiful that when she sang you almost felt you couldna' breathe, and no-one moved a muscle. When they practised their singing I would go along, but the Charge soon learnt how to handle her, and he'd have her singing on her own, or he'd teach her what he called "descants", and she were the star of the whole choir.

But you had to be careful. The poor Superintendent's wife tried to speak to her at the end of one service. I were no longer sitting with her in the choir (I were no singer!). No-one told her not to touch Aggie, and when Aggie looked at the ground and wouldna' look up, she reached out to take her hand, and the screaming... well, it had to be heard to be believed! One of the nurses slapped Aggie, but she shouldn't ha'; it just made her worse. They wouldn't have if Liza had been there. I was glad though, the Superintendent's wife didn't run away, or look frightened or angry, and I saw she stayed to talk to the Charge, while they sent for me and a piece of paper and a pencil, because by now we'd all learnt that the quickest way to calm Aggie down was to let her draw her circles.

So now Aggie had her own role, Liza was busy in the afternoons with the seamstresses, and I was learning to read and write. But I needed more to do. Liza still expected me to look after Ruth when she was not there, but Ruth wouldna' talk with me, and she just made me cross and miserable. Once I even said to her, "Will tha' not stop feelin' sorry for tha'sel'?"

And all she said was, "I am wearisome and a burden to you, Mary, don't bother with me," so what could I do? I just felt shamed.

VIII

I KNEW THERE WERE SUMMAT DIFFERENT IN the air one morning when I woke with the day bell, and the day were already heavy with the summer heat and the promise of thunder. We dressed slowly as if the heat had swaddled us. So it were a shock when one of the ladies shrieked like I'd never heard anyone before, and fell to the floor as stiff as a board. Then she started shaking, and one of the nurses cried, "'Tis the epilepsy, she has the falling sickness, she's having a fit. Come, help me put her on the bed." Some of the ladies just carried on as if it were nothing, but I'd never seen such a thing before and I was shaking mesel', and my own heart were banging in my chest.

They lifted her on to her bed and one of the nurses climbed on top of her and held her down. She called to me to hold her head, and I knelt on the bed, still shaking myself. She looked as though she might die, and I wondered if I should pray for her soul. But she just went on shaking, for ever and ever, I thought she would never stop, and one of the nurses ran off to find one of the doctors. A bit of me felt we weren't doing it right, and we shouldna' be holding her down: at the back of my mind was the thought that Liza would know what to do, but she weren't offering any advice this morning and I couldna' see her anywhere.

I knew a lot of the patients had fits, but most of them were on the back wards, where they were watched all the time, and where there were padded rooms for 'em, as well as for those who were dangerous. The nurses sometimes told us things like this about the back wards, often as much to warn us of what might happen "if we were difficult" and they had to send us there, as anything. There didn't seem to be anything they could do to stop 'em having the fits.

At last the doctor arrived, with another nurse and a big glass syringe (I'd seen one of them before when they'd given Ruth an injection one time), and he stuck the long metal needle in the poor woman's arm, said it was p'raldehyde. Then she stopped shaking and fell asleep, but the smell from the medicine was foul, worse than the smell of the night commodes in the morning, and it hung round the ward all day, as if there were poison in the air. It were a smell I came to hate over the years, more than the earth closets, more than the pig swill, more than anything; not only 'cause it was so foul, but because it always meant someone had been held down and made small in front of the rest of us.

But today I gathered my ducklings, Aggie and Ruth, and led them off to breakfast.

"You mark my words, we're in for a storm," I told them, as I held my head up like I was in charge of 'em, though my knees were still sore from kneeling on the bed.

The nurse watching over us kept jumping up and down, running round the table and looking out the window. "The rain's already started and the sky's turned really dark. Eat your breakfasts quick, we're going to be busy today."

A streak of lightning lit up the room, and, just after, a clap of thunder cracked and bounced off the walls of the great dining hall, making us all jump and shake, rumbling around us and grumbling off like an old man, stealing away out the window and down the road.

Some of the women screamed. Aggie put her hands over her ears.

"Where's Liza? Mary, have you seen her?"

"Where's Liza?"

"She'll not get far in this!"

The nurses didna' hurry often, but now someone was running.

"Come, quick, you must go to the day room," and we did as we were bid, scurrying along like rats as had been spooked by the lightning.

Aggie settled happily to drawing her bubbles in the dim light, as the rain was thrown against the windows; and I sat down to write out some of the words I'd learnt from *Mrs Beeton*: flour, sugar, suet, raisins. I made them into a list; the writing looked pretty on the thick sheet of paper. I looked at it: that would make a good solid boiled pudding. What could I do to make it a bit different, a bit more tasty, like the sweet little puddings the Jewish ladies gave my mother? I rested my head in my hands and stared across the table. In the middle was a great pot of geraniums with bright red flowers, red as blood when you wash it down the sink, not like the wispy pink rose geraniums mother kept on the window sill when I was so very small. She would make tea with the leaves if we couldna' sleep o' night, just a little in a tiny china cup she kept for her babies, and you'd fall asleep, thinking you were out in the warm summer sun and you could smell the dog roses growin' in the hedgerows. Now perhaps there were an idea in this. Could you make a suet pudding with rose geranium? If the flour were leavened a little? Would you taste the roses like you did in the tea?

"This is her day room, ma'am," as the heavy door swung open and Matron swept in. I looked up from my daydreaming. She were a large lady, in the same long-skirted uniform as the nurses but no apron. We didna' see her on our wards much, but when we did she was always frowning. Today her frown seemed to reach down to the corners of her mouth, pinching her lips, and drawing in her cheeks, as the nurses fluttered round her like clothes moths round a candle. She walked round the edge of the room, looking at the windows and the tables and chairs, and then she moved toward me where I were sitting with Aggie. "You can read and write?"

"A little, ma'am, I am learning."

"And who is teaching you?"

"Liza, ma'am."

"Indeed. So this is a list of ingredients. Can you cook?"

"I was a kitchen maid before I came here."

"And what work do you do here?"

"None, ma'am."

"Find her a position in the kitchen then, Charge. The Devil makes work for idle hands!" And then, more softly, to me, "The writing is neat, but look, you have reversed the "s"s. Like this, see? Keep practising, my dear, literacy opens many doors," and then again to the nurses, "Perhaps we should find her a more suitable tutor!"

And with that she swept back out of the room, the door closed, and the key grated in its lock. I looked at Aggie and giggled, but she just reached across me and copied the "s" on my paper. Maybe she could learn to copy other letters as well, instead of drawing circles all the time. Mebbe I could teach her to write her own name, such a pretty name: Agnes Clara.

I looked up to see the other ladies watching me, the only one spoken to by Matron, and I felt my face burning.

"Look 'ee, through the window, the sky's lightening. Perhaps we shall go out to the airing courts soon." But no, we were to spend the rest of the day in the day room.

At bedtime I looked round again for Liza, but she were nowhere to be seen. I asked if t' other ladies had seen her, but no-one remembered seeing her all day. So I asked the nurses, but all they would say was that they "couldn't say". The coat tails of the day's storm were still in the air and the ward was hot and stuffy. We were woken more often than usual by the night nurses unlocking and locking the ward door, and we slept poorly. We did not dare leave our beds, and even Ruth didna' get up.

The next day we rose as usual with the day bell. Emily, who had had the fit, had slept all yesterday, but now she got dressed, though someone had to help her as she was all wobbly on her feet. I think she were hungry, mind, as she had not eaten at all all the day before.

"Ruth, help me wit' blankets." She were just sitting on her bed. She came over and together we folded the blankets, but she didn't say nowt, so I could hear what two of the nurses, standing near and folding blankets as well, were saying.

"They think she went out of the closet window."

"That woulda' been a tight squeeze."

"She's thin and wiry enough though. Probably went before daybreak."

"How did she not fall and break her neck?"

"Mebbe she had a rope."

"And mebbe she grew wings! How could she have got a rope?"

"Who knows."

"P'raps she never came back to the ward. Just walked out."

"Don't let the Charge hear that. They'll say we should have made sure they were all here before locking up."

"Well…"

"Anyway she's been here long enough, knows the place like the back of her hand, she does."

"And she knows everyone, and she's trusted: got a lot of 'em round her little finger, even if they wouldn't dare turn their backs on her."

I realised they were talking about Liza. Had she left then? Just taken herself out of here?

"They say if you're out for fourteen days and you can take care of yourself you can't be mad. Could mean her freedom."

"Her 'usband would never allow that. He sent her here in the first place."

"Didn't she attack him with a knife?"

"Dunno, never heard the full story. Been before the court though."

"If she goes back to Ireland…"

"Back to her sister in Manchester, more like. They'll get her there."

I wanted to ask, but they weren't speaking to me, and I feared they'd be angry. So I tugged at the blanket we were folding, in my own crossness, and it slipped out of Ruth's fingers. Tears filled her eyes and she sat back on the bed behind her and put her hands over her face. I looked at her, then I felt reet mean, so I sat down beside her and put my arm round her.

"I'm sorry, Ruth. I was cross 'cause I don't know where Liza is, and the nurses were talking 'bout her." They had moved away now.

"Liza told me she was going, Mary." Ruth took her hands from her face and stopped sobbing. She spoke very quietly so as I could hardly hear her. "She left with the girls who come in from outside to work in the sewing room. She said they wouldn't tell on her, they like her."

I didn't believe it. "Why didst she tell thee?"

"I don't know. Sometimes when we're walking she tells me things. I don't think she thinks I listen. Sometimes I don't think she's talking to me at all. There are other people… in her head? I don't know. It's like she's in a different world."

I'd seen her as well, talking to herself, as if there were others talking back.

"And I think she had a baby, Mary, once. I don't know what happened to it but she doesn't want to know about my baby at all, not like you."

"But Ruth, I just want my baby so much, and you have yours if you want him."

"I know, Mary, but how can I tell you how this feels? I'm so sorry, Mary, I'm so sorry," and she started sobbing again. She cried and she cried, and how could I be angry with her? I put both my arms round her and tried to stop her crying, but the only thing I could think of to say was, "Come, we must go for breakfast, the nurses are waiting for us, happen we'll have more o' that lovely porridge."

And I did think she smiled, just a little bit.

But it were strange without Liza. She always knew what was what and she made me feel safe. She liked to laugh and joke with the nurses, but she wouldna' let them bully us: I think they were a bit frightened of her. Without her Aggie was more difficult, prickly like a hedgehog, rolling into a ball and screaming whenever anyone came near her, refusing to move from the clock on the corridor wall, arranging and rearranging the food on her plate. And Ruth's pacing up and down the ward at night got worse. We were all jumpy, like fleas on an old dog, and there were more fights among the ladies. And the weather were still hot and the nights thundery, making us itch under our woollen skirts and find fault with everything.

Then happen something cheered me up. One morning, shortly after the day bell had rung, the Charge sought me out. "You're to go to the kitchens today, Mary."

I said to Ruth to keep an eye on Aggie, and then I went with one of the nurses along the corridors toward the dining halls, skipping every few steps with excitement (and to keep up). The dining halls, for there were one for the men and one for the women, were in the big building at the front of the old asylum. It were the building you could see from the road outside. I thought, when I were a child, mebbe that's what a castle looked like. There were a big roadway led from the gates up to the great front doors, and on either side were rose beds. I didn't know what was through those doors, but I knew our dining hall were to one side, as you could see the roadway from the windows.

The nurse took me through the dining hall, down more corridor and into the kitchens. My, they were big, and hot and steamy; and I could see long scrubbed tables, and pans on hooks, and gas cookers like I was used to but much bigger. But I didn't have time to gawp.

"Bin a kitchen maid, have tha'? Well, I'm Cook in charge here. Sit there and clean those 'taties." She pointed to two high stools. On one side were a sack of earthy potatoes and on t' other a pan of water for the clean ones. A lady from one of the other wards was already sitting on one of the stools and working on the potatoes (I knew she were a patient by her clothes, but I noticed there were a few other girls there from "outside" in modern clothes and pinafores, like I'd seen in the *Woman's Weekly*. And they looked like they were my age as well). Cook gave me a knife to peel with. "Clean, mind, peel only if tha' has to, and look sharp. Just because I'm soft and let thee sit doesna' mean tha' can go to sleep."

I settled down to my work; I wanted to skip and dance around the room. This was work I was used to, and the potatoes smelt of the good fresh soil they'd come from. After a while, though, I did wish there were something else I could do: the skin on my fingers was getting all wrinkly, and every potato was just like the last one. I smiled at the lady beside me, but she said nowt.

At last Cook came over and took a look at our work. "Mind tha' don't take too much potato wi' t' peel." She was a tall woman, with large hands, and feet in clogs. But she moved fast, as I soon learnt to my cost. She had a bird-like face with a sharp nose and sharp brown eyes, and her head seemed to be moving all the time, tipping to one side to see better, like a blackbird with a worm, and if she saw you doing something wrong, or idlin', there'd be a slap in it for you, that suddenly came out of nowhere, and was oft measured out wi' a wooden spoon. She kept order in her kitchen, but she weren't cruel.

"What's tha' name?"

"Well, Mary. I knows every woman who works in here, and what their work is like; and I knows the name of each and every one of 'em. If tha' works well for me I'll not mither thee, but if not… well, tha'll soon be walking the airing courts all day again. And I'll not stand for thieving neither. Tha'll be fed well and have no need of tastin' else."

"And no chatting, neither," added my companion.

"Ay, and I heard that, and she's right. Chattin's for soldiers in trenches with lice in their pants, not for the likes of thee and me. Now finish those potatoes." And she turned away.

I smiled across the potatoes. "I'm Dorothy." Now my fellow potato peeler spoke. "I once cooked for the queen, you know!"

My heart sank. Which queen?

"Victoria, of course!"

I knew other ladies on our ward who would tell strange stories like this. You had to be careful. Sometimes they believed they knew who you were, or they heard voices telling them about you, oft-times not nice things, so they might be frightened of you, or try to hurt you. But Dorothy seemed quite calm, and no-one else was at all upset by her, so I stopped worrying. But I took mind of the "No chatting" order, and kept my peace, carrying on with the potatoes, and Dorothy spoke no more.

When we'd cleaned the potatoes we had to chop them and add them to the great stew pans. Then we had breakfast. True to her word Cook made sure we had plenty of porridge, and we were each allowed a teaspoonful of honey with it, a treat for sure. "The bees has done us proud this year gone, plenty of honey to last through," she commented.

After dinner and we'd cleaned and cleared we were lined up and our aprons checked for stowed knives. Then we were taken back to join t' others from our wards in the airing courts. I was jumpin' to tell Ruth and Aggie, and anyone else who would listen, about the kitchens and about my working there, but no-one cared to hear. So I fell in with Aggie, and, walking round and round, I told her my tales, though I knowed they were falling on deaf ears.

The following days I was taken from the ward before the day bell had rung: one of the nurses would bid me rise and dress, and then lead me down the long tiled corridors to the kitchen. I had more time then to look around me: there were old coke ovens as well as the gas-fired ones, and gas hobs, and pots and pans for an army. I suppose it *were*, to be true, like feeding an army: there must have been nigh on a doubled thousand o' bellies to fill in the hospital, and they were all filled from here. Using my new arithmetic I had worked out that there were more 'n five hundred women came for their meals in our dining hall alone.

There were big store rooms and a larder, and a meat room where they brought the animals killed from the farm, and where they butchered 'em and hung 'em, and weighed all the meat before it came into the kitchen. And there were great sinks, and a smaller kitchen as well with a modern range; that was where they cooked the food for the doctors and any visitors, and it was where the first electric cooker were put. We had electric lights in the day room, but none on the wards (only the old gas lights), but here there were lots, so even in the dark days of winter you could see what you were doing.

It were always hot and busy in there, but I didna' mind. There must have been more 'n two dozen patients working there, all women, you could tell 'em by their clothes, but there were the girls from "outside" as well. We were collected each morning from the wards and brought here to put together breakfast, after which we could eat ourselves, and then we had to prepare the midday meal, our main meal, and after that our tea. We ate our dinner after the rest of the patients, and washed up and then they took us back to our wards or day rooms, or to the airing courts. We did this oft-times six or seven days a week. The food was simple, nothing fancy like, mainly stews and porridge, but we baked bread as well, and there were often stewed fruit, mostly rhubarb and windfall apples, and even, if we were really lucky, eggs. It filled us up well. Wherever possible, I learnt, the food came from the hospital farm and the kitchen gardens, and nothing were wasted. Summer plenty was bottled and salted and preserved for winter. Some of the work I was used to, but I were soon learning new things as well.

Then, one evening when we were taken back to our ward, Liza was there. It were about ten days after she'd gone, and she were lying on her bed. She were asleep and I couldna' rouse her, but I guessed she had put up a fight when they'd found her, as the smell of the p'raldehyde was hanging on her. (They used the p'raldehyde for calmin' a body down if they couldna' cope wi''em, as well as for the fits.) Her hair was all untidy and her eyes had black rings around them.

In the morning I had to leave for my kitchen work before she woke, so I couldna' speak to her till the afternoon in the airing courts. Her walk along the paths was more of a shuffle, as if she'd fall any minute, and she wouldna' look at me. I put my arm through hers, but she took it away, and drew her shawl more tightly round her shoulders.

"I'm glad to see you again, Liza, are you feeling better?" I asked.

She said nowt for a while.

"I would ha' thought, to be sure, tha' wouldst ha' done better wi' out me." Her voice was deep and hoarser than usual, and she spoke so soft I could hardly hear her.

"I feel better when you're here, Liza, you make the days pass quicker, and you help me and you answer my questions."

"Well, there's a strange thing for you."

We walked a few more paces. "Can I hold your hand, Liza?"

"If you must, child."

I took her hand and stroked the back of it. The skin was dry and wrinkled like an old woman's, though Liza was not so old. They said that was what the lye soap did to your hands.

She stumbled on the path and my hand tightened on hers. "Are ye not well, Liza, did they hurt you? Why did they give you the p'raldehyde?"

"No questions, child, I am tired, too tired to answer you. There seems no end to this black tunnel we're in. Surely, I could walk on the rails and welcome the train."

I waited a while, but still I wanted to know.

"Where did you go, Liza?"

She sighed, but then she did answer me. I had thowt she mightn't.

"I thought if I could find my sister I could be staying wi' her, but that's where they came for me. He told 'em where I'd be. There'll be no escape 'less I can get to Ireland. Walk, child."

"But will he not speak for you, your husband?"

"Jesus, no, not him. Spent my money and got another woman, 'e 'as. Though she'll soon find what he's like when he's soaked. That's why I'm here, lass. He wanted me here."

"But he…"

"You wanted my story so you might as well have it. He couldn't hold on to a job when he came back from the war. Would go out drinking, and after… he'd want his way with me. And I'd fight him. We were saving for our little guesthouse, we'd both been in service, done all right really. No children, I'd made sure of that, thanks to Marie Stopes." She laughed. "But then he started drinking our savings, and I'd fight him when I caught him a' takin' the money. So he told them I took a knife to him. He told them I said I was ta'en by the Devil. He showed them bruises and cuts, said I'd done them. Said I was mad, and they believed him. Said I couldn't help myself. Said I heard voices. I'll say I heard voices, my own, screaming some sense into him! And sure, I took a knife to warn him off. Bruises from his fists would have cost me my job. You couldn't have a housekeeper with a black eye, now, could ye?

"And I screamed and kicked when they took me, so they put me in a padd, and every time they opened the door I fought like a cat for my freedom, till I saw that was just what they expected. Then I thought I could show 'em it was all lies by being good and doing as they wanted, but that didn't help neither. Couldn't see any way out but through the closet window, but, mercy, those windows are small! But I found a way." She allowed herself a small smile at this and I saw a glimmer of the old Liza in it. But her voice was weary and her hands shook as she spoke.

"I thought you walked out wi' the girls from the village?" I whispered so the nurses wouldn't hear me.

"Hush now, there's more 'an one way to skin a rabbit. But, ye know, I loved him once," her voice drifted away, "and, to be sure, we had a great dream, but men were never meant to live like rats in tunnels, and be shot and gassed, and kill, and die in agony together."

"And your baby? Ruth said…"

"Babies are the work of the Devil." Her voice came back loud and strong again. "I've told 'ee: no talk of babies."

And with that she took her hand out of mine and turned away to sit on a bench, where she rocked herself, to and fro, like Aggie often did. And I was frightened of asking more or putting my arm round her as I might have done another. So I let her alone and found Aggie to walk with, and I put what she'd told me away in my mind to think on sometime else.

IX

SLOWLY LIZA WERE TURNED BACK INTO THE Liza I knew. She grew strong and stood straight again, and she scolded us and chivvied us, and made us laugh, and the sameness of every day laid a little less heavy on us. The hardness would still come back into her eyes, though, when she thought you weren't watching, and I was still afeared of telling her my kitchen stories.

Then one day Ruth were taken away and I asked Liza if she knew what was to be done with her.

"Happen I do, Mary. 'Tis usual with the melancholia. She will go to the infirmary; I heard one of the nurses say she is to have the sleeping treatment. They will give her a draught to keep her asleep for most of the day and night for five days or so, just waking her to eat and wash. Sometimes it helps."

"Will it help Ruth?"

"Who knows." Liza's voice was quiet. "Surely I hope and pray it does, for she doesn't deserve this. And neither do you, "Oh Little Friend of All the World". Tomorrow you will tell me of your kitchen adventures and we shall be friends again."

I was glad of that but the bed seemed extra hard that night and I couldn't lie comfie. When at last I slept, I dreamt my mother was sitting beside me peeling potatoes. Then I woke early, and lay in the dark, thinking on what I should do. Mebbe I would ask Liza to help me write a letter to my mother. Could I remember the name of the last house where we had worked, and the street it were in? Perhaps then she would speak for me and I could leave this place. But I was troubled: I would miss Aggie, and I had a job now in the kitchens. It was safe here. Mostly I knew what to expect. Mebbe, though, I'd be able to find my baby. I thought of him less these days. I couldn't see him in my mind growing, laughing, learning to crawl and blowing bubbles like as baby Sam did. I could only think of him as a tiny little thing with a wrinkled nose and suckling mouth, soft and warm and pink in my arms, and that memory itself was like an age away now. But when I did think of him I still hurt inside for him, like a bit of me had been cut out with one of Cook's kitchen knives, and there were a hole left behind and an emptiness I thought would be with me for ever.

My arm was shaken. "Hurry, or you'll be late, and Cook won't stand for lateness." I dressed quickly and, led by the nurse, joined the other sleepyheads, yawning, rubbing their eyes, slop slopping down to the kitchens.

"Good morning, Dorothy."

"'Mornin', sweetheart."

I smiled at them. I was pleased, I had a plan. But the faces kept turned from me, or just glanced quick at me. Some were in their own worlds far away from the rest of us, and some grumpy at being woken so early. I would not be afeared of Dorothy, I decided, and I *would* write to my mother. But now I would settle to the day's work: more vegetables to clean and chop, sweet young carrots and turnips today. So, standing at the long table, its boards scrubbed white from its cleaning,

I scraped and chopped and thought how I would write my letter.

When the day was done I couldn't wait to get back to the ward to tell Liza my plan, dancing along the corridors and running up the stairs, even though the nurses were sharp with me, but when at last I could tell her she did not think well of it. "I will help you, but they may not let you send a letter, and you have no money for the postage. Then they may read the reply and you may not be allowed to see it. I have tried to write to my sister."

"But, Liza, I can remember the name of the house and the street it were in."

We were getting ready for bed and it were still difficult to talk to her, which made me cross. Her bed were some way from mine and the nurses were telling us not to dawdle. They wanted to get us settled and locked in so they had time for themselves.

I folded my day clothes and placed them under my bed, then I climbed in and took the doll from under my pillow. "We will find Peter, we will," I whispered, "and he shall play with you. I shall help him build a house for thee from sticks and stones, and I will make thee some clothes if we can find some scraps and a needle an' thread. And I will teach Peter as Liza teaches me, so he can read and write."

The door slammed shut, the keys jangling on their ring, and the nurses had gone. Liza came to my bedside.

"We will write your letter tomorrow afternoon in the day room."

"And shall we tell me ma where I am? Perchance she don't know. Then she can come an' get me."

"Surely we will."

"I can ask the nurses to sharpen my pencil and I can write it on one of the last pieces of the butcher's block paper. You can help me with the spellings and how to set the writing out."

"But you must sleep now, child. I fear you will be sorely hurt by this plan of yours, so temper your hope with patience, little friend. Goodnight."

And the next afternoon she did help me, and I wrote my neatest writing and we gave it to the Charge; and when I saw Molly I asked if it would be posted, and she smiled at me, and teased me, for who could I be writing letters to, and I told her it was to me mother, and she said she would make sure it was posted for me.

Then all I could do was wait to see what would happen.

*

I carried on working in the kitchens and each day began to fall into a pattern. Day in, day out, nothing changed.

Then, nearly a week later, Ruth came back to us.

Liza took her arm and steadied her as she walked round the airing court. "You must get your strength back, my dear." And Ruth smiled at her.

"You still look tired, Ruth. What was it like? Sleeping all day?" I had to ask her, I had to know. "And do you feel better?"

"It was very tiring." She laughed quietly. I'd not heard her laugh before, it were such a soft sound I hardly heard it then. "But I don't remember much. Now I think I want to see my baby, so does that mean I'm better? I'd like to go home... perhaps. My poor husband..."

She looked past me as if she could see something over my shoulder.

But then she looked at me again. "You know, I have a beautiful little house, with beautiful furniture, and carpets, and damask bedlinen, and here I am walking round a courtyard all day and sleeping in a prison. I *must* be mad!"

"And did ye have pretty clothes, and a maid to put them out for you, and a cook to cook your food?"

"No, Mary, my husband is only an articled clerk, and we don't have a great deal of money. We have a housekeeper who comes in to clean and do the washing for us each day, but I have had to learn to cook for us. The bedlinen and the furniture were my dowry. But I do have some pretty clothes, not like these great heavy things we have to wear in here."

"And does your house have a garden, and will you grow roses, and will your little boy run on the grass and hide in the trees?"

"Jesus, Mary, you'll drive us all to an early grave with your questions." Liza was smiling as well. "Now let us all rightly be glad we have Ruth back, and not speak of the future. Come, Ruth, take no mind of her." And there seemed something between them I couldna' be part of, so I left them and I walked with Aggie.

But if it were good news for Ruth, the fact that she were a bit better could not help me feel good when I got my letter back. The Charge handed it me one morning on my way to the kitchens. It had been put in an envelope and redirected "return to sender". I turned it over, and with my finger I traced the words as I read what was written on the back: "Mrs Pearson left our employ before Christmas 1926 and was taken to the workhouse infirmary, where we understand she passed away."

The Charge must've read those words as well, but she said nowt but, "Don't keep Cook waiting; you have work to do."

So I put the letter in my apron and followed the nurse to the kitchen, where I did as I was bid and got on with my work. I kept feeling for the letter in my apron. I could not believe what it said. It was wrong. I would read it again and see it was wrong. Liza would show me the mistake.

But at the end of the day's working when I saw Liza in the airing court she said it looked correct to her. But she were gentle with me and she said we would speak to the Charge and find out more, and I must not fret as she must have been very poorly from the chemicals, and surely it must have been a blessed relief to her.

And we walked together quietly for a while, till I saw Molly come through the door. She came straight over to me and her face was very red and she were breathing hard.

"What right did you have to write that letter, Mary? What right did you have to bother God-fearing people with your worries about your ailing mother? If I had known what you were doing I would have stopped the letter from being posted."

I didn't know what to say. I thought I would cry, but I wasna' going to... she was being unfair. But Liza stepped between us. "She had every right. Jesus, can a woman no make a civil enquiry of another... or is she getting above her station?"

"She is a mental hospital patient; what anxiety has she caused to an innocent family?"

"Mebbe she's pricked their consciences?"

"That is not her place."

"Nor is it yours to interfere."

"And this is your doing as well, Liza, you watch your step. We hear your whisperings... to the nurses, to the girls who come in to work here, yes, even to the patients. Your talk of unions and equality, women's rights. You are dangerous and you'll get your comeuppance one day."

"One day the working men and women of this country will rise up against the likes of you, with your fancy houses, your servants, and your money, made on the backs of others, and, Jesus, Mary and Joseph, we'll not lock up women like this as needs our care."

"Mind what you say, Liza. I will not tolerate this insolence!"

"What will ye do? Remember, I'm a patient. Ye'll be dismissed if ye hit me. Surely I'll no hide the bruises."

"I'll not forget this, Liza, mark my words."

"Well, I say, what will you do? Will you tell 'Daddy'? And will he no give his money to keep the 'undeserving' out of sight and off the streets, and will he tell them in Parliament of the insubordination and ingratitude of the patients in the mental hospitals?"

"I will listen to no more of this, but you will pay for this, Liza. You may be clever, but I have power and wealth and generations of leadership on my side. That will break the strikes and make Britain great again. That will restore the proper order of things again. That will ensure people like you don't grow too big for your boots."

Then she turned and walked, or even ran perhaps, out of the airing court again. And Liza squeezed my hand. "Take no notice, Mary, she had no right to speak to you like that."

But that were no comfort, and when I went to bed I cried and I cried, softly mind, under the covers, and with the old doll clutched to my chest, the metal hooks digging in me. And I thought on me ma again, pretty as she was, before she worked in the factories, like an angel from a picture in her Bible, dancing round the room with Sam in her arms. But it was me she kept when she had no money, and the boys she took to the Children's Village. She always made me safe, and sometimes she hid me away. Should I have cared for her more? Did I not know she were that poorly? I think I did me best. Liza says I'm just a child. But I'm not. Mebbe I don't know much of the world, but I can learn. Even in this place I can learn. And I will learn.

She didna' say much to me those last days, me ma; she were too tired and she coughed too much. She never said what would happen when the baby came, and I never thowt to ask.

We'd get by, like always, the two of us, just with the baby as well.

Did she know she were dying? Is that why she left me at the workhouse? Was that always what she was going to do?

I think she loved me, though she never said, but she were part o' me, and I miss her, and she never said goodbye.

In the morning I stayed under the covers till Liza came. "You must be getting up, Mary. Come, wash your face, get dressed. Go to the kitchens and I will ask the Charge what became of your mother."

"She should've told me she were dying. Why did she not tell me?"

"There are many as cannot say they're dying, even if they know it. Happen your mother couldn't face that you'd be on your own wi' out her, child."

"But I'm not a child, Liza."

"Mebbe… this place makes children of us all. There was a Russian wrote a great book. He said, the strongest of all warriors are these two, Time and Patience. Take hold o' them, Mary, you're young: learn and grow with them beside ye, and may the Mother of God make them that have power o'er us see you should not be here. The greatest enemy in here is the sameness… fight it. Ask a new question every day, and seek the answer. Never give up."

"But what of you, Liza? They say you've seen plenty o' years here."

"I have more to fight than you, my dear, for there be those against me in here and out, and in me own head. I've waged a war against them since I were seventeen, and mostly I've won, but rightly ye won't understand. So be ye not worrying 'bout me. Remember, you are you, believe in yourself, you exist, learn and grow, learn and grow, you are not just another lunatic'. They can only destroy you if you let them. Now just go to the kitchens and work."

So I did, and Cook let me alone to pod peas and string beans in a corner where it were quiet, and I think she must have known as she didn't mither me. But then after a while she set me to making pastry. "Pies make everything go further, Mary. Mark my words, flour and lard and water fills a few bellies, and tha hands are cold for it."

She didn't need to teach me, but it were hard work making that much pastry: my arms would ache with the rolling of it. And every little scrap had to be used. If there were any left I'd cut shapes of leaves or berries or flowers and put them on the tops of the pies or pasties before I brushed 'em with water, and it'd make Cook mad. "Tha didst na' come here to waste time on fancies, missy." But she laughed the day I fashioned a mouse's backside and a long curly tail coming outta roly-poly pudding. And I laughed as well, and it were good to laugh again.

And back in the airing courts Ruth was laughing more as well. And eating her food better. So it weren't long before they sent her home. But before she went she talked with me.

"You and I, Mary, we're from different worlds. I probably have more in common with Aggie, and certainly I do with Liza, who is an educated woman, than I do with you. But lately you have been kind to me and I am grateful. I know you find it hard to understand how I could abandon my baby, but I think I can understand your unhappiness better than you can mine. It's just difficult for me to show that I care when I am constantly worrying about what will happen to me and to my baby. You know, my biggest fear is that there will be another war. It's more than ten years since the last one and I should have forgotten it by now, but I still wake at night hearing the knock on the door coming to tell my mother that another of my brothers is dead. How could we bring babies into a world with so much strife, Mary? What future is there for them?"

I knew she were older than me, but I didn't like her setting herself above me, though I knew she were right. I were just a working girl with no learnin', and she had a husband with a real job, and a house and nice clothes. But I were cross with her that she couldn't see a life for our babies. And I were sad as well, for there was still that look in her eyes, as though she were looking through us all at summat far away. She were still not well, to my mind.

Liza came up to us. "Take care, Ruth. Be strong. You're as good as any man out there, and sure, don't you be forgettin' that." She smiled.

"And, Mary, the Charge has found out a bit more for us about your mother. She did indeed die in the workhouse, of bronchitis and yellow jaundice from the chemicals."

I felt as if she'd hit me in the belly. "I should ha' been with her. Where is her body now?"

"She had a pauper funeral, and she will ha' been buried in a pauper grave, but the Charge didna' know where."

I bit my lip and tried not to cry, and all that silly woman, Ruth, says to me is, "I will pray for her, Mary, and for your baby."

I wanted to hit her, I wanted to throw her prayers back in her face: how could she care so little? But Liza took my hand and squeezed it. "You are growing stronger, Mary, and now you are reading better I have asked the Charge for more books for the day room, so as you can practise on more than recipes and the *Woman's Weekly*. You can learn much from books."

"Won't bring my baby back."

"But might help you to find him. I ha' told ee, look at the ladies around ye: every day they get up, get dressed, go dine, walk. Mindless days, day in day out the same, till they can't think of nowt else. You must fight it, fight the sameness, fight the shrinking of the warp and the weft, fight for your future, Mary, for you have one… and learnin' and books'll help."

"Not helped yet."

"Have patience. Your time will come."

"But what of you? Have you read books, Liza?"

"Indeed I have. There was a free library in Dundalk, where I grew up. I wasn't allowed to take books home, but the librarian was sweet on my mother's young sister, and he would turn a blind eye to me in a corner of the reading room. I were one of twelve, so my mother was happy for me to be out of the way. My father loved the books, no doubt, but he was but a stevedore, and with so many mouths to feed he had neither time nor money for reading. But he wanted his children to do better, and he liked nothing more than to hear me tell the stories I'd read by the fire of a night.

"He were a good man, my father: though there were twelve of us he taught us we were each valued and special, made us strong, gave us the fight in our bellies.

"As soon as I could leave school, though, I went into service. But I were a good accountant, and I kept a little money back from my wage each week and saved it. The rest they needed at home. And then I met William, and we married and travelled to England, where there were more opportunities, and together we worked and saved… till the call-up for the Great War spoilt everything. But through all that time I never stopped reading, you could always find a free library somewhere."

"And you can escape into exciting foreign countries, and the exotic worlds of the imagination in books, Mary," Ruth joined in.

"And will us learn new words like that?" I sniffed.

"Tha' will that, lass," laughed Ruth. And I laughed as well; mebbe Ruth wasn't that bad; her teasing and her prayers were meant well.

"But your reading's not got *you* out of here, Liza!"

"Nor will it, as long as they plot against me."

"Who, Liza?"

"Never you mind. They come from the very gates of Hell. Sure, this is the Devil's paradise here, but you do not belong. Neither surely does Ruth. But do your own growing and you will get out."

So Ruth went, and the Charge found us old copies of books by Charles Dickens and Jane Austen, and by Kipling, (I loved the tales of Kim and Mowgli) but she also found us some books I found more difficult, like *War and Peace*, and volumes of poetry, as well. Sometimes Liza would read me poems and I loved to hear the rhythm of the verses as she read them in her Irish lilt, while I struggled still with spelling out the longer words and finding their meanings. And Aggie would join us and listen, and then you'd hear her saying lines, word for word, to herself later. I never could understand how she could do this and yet never speak to us. But I did love her for it.

And somehow I knew Liza was right: words would save me. In the end my learnin', my reading and my writing, would answer my questions, and I *would* grow up.

X.

DAY BY DAY I GREW TO LIKE MY WORK MORE
and more. We were mighty busy in that kitchen, but
it were good to be busy, and though it were hot and
steamy and always full o' the noise of pots and pans and lids
and choppin', I loved it.

I grew to like Dorothy's company as well, though never
sure who she would be that day, and whether her stories were
true or not. Often there were a grain of truth to them. Cook
told me she were kitchen maid in Town Hall in Manchester
when Queen Victoria came to open the Ship Canal, but
whether or not she really cooked for the Queen I couldna' tell.
But she were harmless, and she were strong, the kind of help
you needed when the storerooms had to be cleared, as they
oft did because of the rats, who nibbled their way through the
storage sacks, despite all the cats that came in to hunt them.
The cats were wild, but Cook called them in with scraps,
and they certainly worked hard. Cook kept an 'edgehog an'
all, to eat the beetles, and the other creepie-crawlies, and the
bleached yellow slugs that came out from the drains at night.

But he slept through winter, and I swear he carried as many bugs on him as he ate.

But making so many meals was hard work. Cook divvied up the duties for the day and put us in "sections" with one of the girls from "outside" over each section (though often they knew less about what needed to be done than us!). She kept a special eye out for me and would send me off to do things on me own for her. "Take tha'sel off and make me three dozen 'tatie pasties. Quick, mind, they're needed for the farm workers. Not too much meat, mind, or they'll think I've gone soft on 'em."

And I'd set to, and crimp the edges, and prick them, and use the scrapings of leftover pastry to make 'em pretty, and glaze them with water, and all in double quick time, and she'd come over and "tut" at me and ask me where I got my airs and graces from, but I could see she was proud of 'em when they came out the oven and she passed them to the men as came to the door.

"I were a mill girl mesel'," she'd say. "I know a man works better on a full stomach."

Time passed, then one evening when we were back to the ward for our beds we found Ruth with us again, curled up on a bed, her face to the wall. She did not answer when I spoke to her and her eyes looked through me as if I weren't there. Then in the night she were up again walking up and down, up and down.

The next day in the airing courts I asked her how her baby was.

"I could not say."

"But you've been with him."

"Don't bother me. His father loves him."

"Is he not growing?"

Her face were pale and she were thin again. I couldna' make her smile.

"We were better dead, he and I."

"But he's your own."

"Go away, Mary, I can't listen to you."

I thought mebbe I could make her feel better so I put my arm around her, but she turned away and shrugged me off. I thought mebbe if we talked of summat else…

"I go to the kitchen near every day now, Ruth. I made pasties for the farm workers t'other day." But she didn't seem interested.

So I knew her sister were looking after her baby when she could not and I asked her, "And is your sister well? She has a baby of her own an' all, don't she? Will be good for the two little 'uns to grow up together." We had sat on a bench and she pulled her shawl close round her shoulders.

"I had two sisters once. The other died with my mother of the influenza after the war." Then the tears rolled down her cheeks and my heart ached for her sadness, but there were nothing I could do, so I just sat beside her and kept my peace.

And after a while her sobbing quieted and she started to talk as she'd not done to me before. "I had two sisters and three brothers. Two of my brothers died on the Front, but one came back to us. He had lost both his legs and his shoulder was shattered. He was in great pain all the time. Mary, it was terrible. He would scream with it in bed at night. They wouldn't let me near him. All I could hear were the screams. Then one morning they said he had gone. I think he must have taken his life. They never told me. They thought I was just a child, I shouldn't know about these things.

"But that wasn't as bad as my sister. My mother caught the Spanish 'flu and coughed and fevered till she just gave up. But my sister, I can never forget my sister. She coughed and she couldn't breathe, and every breath she tried to take made her chest hiss and rattle like a boiling kettle, and it was as if she was drowning. And she could hardly speak but her eyes were wide as if she was really frightened. And, Mary, I was with her when she died. All on my own. I'd said I'd watch her. And she tried to sit up, and she couldn't speak, and her eyes were asking me to help her, wide and staring from her face with the fear of it, and I couldn't do anything. She tried to fight it, and I couldn't help her. And I'll see her eyes begging me to help her till the day I die. And I'll hear that sound of her drowning... I wake at night sometimes and she's there and I can't help her. And I can't breathe then myself, for she's dying again and I have done nothing."

"But what could you have done, you but a child y'self?"

She didna' answer me. She wasn't crying any more. It were as if she'd cried herself out. She just sat and stared at her hands and I couldna' rouse her.

And then she would not move when they said it were time to go to the dining hall. One of the nurses twisted her arm to make her stand up and she cried out. Then Liza came out of nowhere and took hold o' the nurse's arm and twisted that till *she* cried out, and two more nurses came and shouted at Liza that she'd be for the "padd" if she didn't watch out, and before you could say "Jack Robinson" there were ladies fighting the nurses and ladies fighting ladies, and Ruth were just sat in the middle of it. But it didn't last for long. Some of the ladies just liked an excuse for pulling hair and scratching, and it were soon over, and Liza was good at calming things down anyway, and she took Ruth's hand, her head in the air, and they walked to the dining hall as if nothing had happened, and everyone followed, with the nurses straightening their caps and aprons and muttering about telling the Charge. (That were funny, they were so discomfited, but I didn't dare laugh; but Aggie did, though I don't know why. I didn't think she'd even noticed the fighting.)

Then it were not long after that they took Ruth away. "Gone for the new electric shock treatment," the nurses said. And nothing more happened to Liza, though the nurses kept well away from her.

So I just kept on with my kitchen work, till one day, "Goodness gracious!" Cook was put out: one of the doctors had come to the kitchen. She bustled him away, and came back to me.

"He's heard of some new-fangled diet to treat them 'leptics, stop their fits. Come, Mary, you can do this, I've no time for it."

I was getting to know Cook's cooking were simple and basic. She made sure the kitchens produced solid, filling food for us all. She were good at organising us, and she knew every bit of what was going on. But changes to her routines upset her. "I'm not unreasonable, but I cannot be doing wi' doctors in t' kitchens."

He was a young doctor I'd not seen before, not that we saw much of the doctors anyway. He was sat at a table in one of the store rooms, his starched collar looking to weep in the steam from the boiling vegetables, and his chin on his hand. He sat up. "Matron said she had spoken to you, Mrs Bradshaw."

"She has indeed. Tell what you want to this lass, she'll do it."

"The superintendent has given me leave to treat three of our epileptic patients with a special diet. In some cases the diet has been shown to reduce the number of seizures they suffer. It has the same effect as starvation, only they're not to be starved but fed a great deal of fat, and very little carbohydrate or protein. Do you know what that means?"

"No, sir."

"I have been working with one of the nurses, Miss Turner, in the infirmary. We have been given an outline of the main constituents of the patients' daily diet, and we have examined it. Can you read?"

"Mostly, sir."

"Well, we have listed here all those constituents under their nutritional nature as fat; protein: things like meat; or carbohydrate: sugar and starch. Our patients must have no less than four times as much fat in what they eat as the other foods. I have taken advice from others who have instituted this treatment, and I have done some calculations myself and this is an example of a menu. It is critical that you adhere to the regime. Miss Turner and I have taken into account the foods available to you and we think this is possible. Do you understand?"

I looked at the diet sheet. It didn't seem to make much sense. I studied it hard and out of the muddle of words a thread began to appear: very little meat or potatoes, everything fried in butter, lots of cream. It made me feel quite ill.

"You must do this just as it says." He had put his chin on his hand again, but though his words sounded very posh I thought he were a touch frightened of me. "We have to know that you are following the diet correctly. You must write down each day exactly what you prepare for these patients. You mustn't let us down."

"I will do my best, sir."

"Everything must be weighed. Can you do that?" He were beggin' me!

"We've learnt her some arithmetic. She'll manage."

"And record the weights?"

I swallowed. My mouth was dry. What if I made a mistake?

Nowt was said for a while then he asked if we had any questions, and whether we were not satisfied with what he had said, and when we still said nowt he stood up.

But then he stopped and turned back to us. "If we could find a cure for these patients... They have a hard life. They are shunned by their families. There are many who say we should sterilise them all, operate on them to stop them fathering more tainted individuals. It's a cruel world.

"If they didn't have the fits, the falling attacks, they might not be in here.

"So your work is important."

Then he left, and we were left with his lists. At least he cared. And what about me? What was my "cure"?

But Cook just grumbled. "Not natural. Shouldna' interfere with nature. Where will I get all that cream from? 'Tis meant for the butter. If we was meant to eat cream like that the Lord would ha' given us udders. Take your lists and make what sense you can of them, and don't forget we have two thousand other mouths to feed as well."

I sat for a little longer staring at the sheets of paper. What had Liza said? Ask a new question every day and find the answer: that's the way to stop your mind from not knowing how to think for itself in here. Well, plenty of questions today, and how many new words? Carbo-whats? And I'd have to get quicker with me addin'.

I was frightened I'd get it all wrong, but the next day I started. I put together the meals for the three unknown bodies in the infirmary as set out on the sheets the doctor had left, and I did my best to make them look and taste good to eat. But I was glad I didn't have to eat them, and, though they left the kitchen piping hot, I wondered what they were like when the pools of butter and lard cooled and went hard before they could reach the ward.

It were not a surprise then when the doctor came back to the kitchen one day. "The patients won't eat the food you prepare for them. How can we make it more appetising?"

We sat in the storeroom together and looked at the lists of the meals I had prepared. It was only a small wooden table we sat at, and this time Cook didn't stay with us, so as he put the papers down and we bent over them his head touched mine, and I couldna' help but shiver. I don't think I'd ever been this close to a real man before. He smelt nice as well.

But I was just a kitchen maid, so I told him how I added parsley and rosemary, and rhubarb juice to cut across the lard, but I could do nothing about hot things going cold, or, as much, cold ones warming. "And I would find it hard mesel' to eat the amount that's put to a plate!"

Cook joined us. "You must take the food to the patients tha'sel'. That will make sure it gets there hot, and you can see for yourself what else might help."

I could feel my heart beating in my chest. I was to take the food. Cook was sending me off on my own, trusting me, and to a men's ward an' all. The next day then, though she did send one of the nurses with me, I took the meals I had put together to the infirmary. We took trays and carried them past the kitchen garden and the cricket ground. The three patients were all men, kept in the infirmary, but able to dress and spend the day out of bed. I was sad to see them, they looked poorly and I could see scars and cuts and bruises, old and new, from when the fits took them. They were dull-eyed and little interested in me or the food I brought. They ate a little of it and then turned their backs upon it. I asked what would make it better for them, but they wouldna' speak. I went back to the kitchens and thought I would cry. I could be a good cook, I knew it, but I couldn't make a meal like this as a man would eat.

But I enjoyed my daily walks to the infirmary, and I thought p'rhaps I'd see Ruth if I kept my eyes open. Then one day the nurse there was Molly.

"Molly, we've not seen thee for such a time." Her golden hair was still very carefully curled and pinned and she were as "comfortable" as ever, but she never seemed to stop moving.

The twinkle had gone from her eyes, though, and I couldna' forget her crossness the last time I'd seen her. I though she were a bit wary o' me as well.

"Hello, Mary. I've been working on these diets with Dr Campbell. We have so many patients with epilepsy in here. It would be a major advance if we could stop their seizures. They say starving them helps but we can't do that, so we need to find a way of getting them to eat the food you prepare. Here's the doctor." When he came in her face lifted as if this were the most important thing that could be happening in the world. "Come, sit at this table. Let's discuss this." They put their heads together and cut me out of their talk, of "research" and "papers" and "outcomes". And then, as if it were my fault, Molly looked straight in my face for the first time and shook my menus at me. "Why will they not eat?"

"I dunno. Mebbe I could grind up some nuts as flour, like the charcoal burner said you could do with beechnuts, so we could thicken the sauces, and mebbe if they didn't have to eat so much at each meal?"

"If they had five small meals a day instead of three big ones?"

"All the wards have their own kitchens, mostly no longer in use since the food has come from the central galley, but what if the infirmary kitchen were recommissioned for this project?"

"I could cook them meals that were hot when they got 'em, and mebbe one meal could be a soup, with vegetables off your list as doesn't have too much sugar?"

Molly were excited, I could tell, but she still wouldna' smile at me. My doctor did though, and then he winked at me. My face felt on fire, but all Molly said were, "You're a silly girl, sometimes, Mary." Then I caught the look on her face and she were real angry with me, just for a minute, then she went back to her papers and her plans.

I sat with my hands in my lap. I wanted to cry. What had I done wrong?

"We might get some results worth publishing," Molly was saying, "but let's see if we can arrange the re opening of the infirmary kitchens first."

So I went with Cook, Molly and the doctor to see Matron to ask if we could use the ward kitchen. Now that were a bother, traipsing along all them corridors, the four of us, and waiting outside her "Office". I were scared, but I didn't have to say owt, and it were worth it 'cause a "trial period" was agreed. I would go every day to the infirmary to cook for "my" three patients, and if what I cooked was eaten I would teach the nurses on the ward the recipes.

Every morning I was taken to the kitchen and then to the infirmary, where I spent the rest of the day. I always had a nurse with me, but the walk each day were good, and I liked to see "my" patients. After their coldness to me on that first day, they began to get used to me, and then they would greet me at least with a word, but sometimes with a smile as well. Some days they would be sleeping after fits, or smelling of the dread p'raldehyde, or they'd have fresh cuts and bruises from falling in an attack. They couldn't see much point in the diet, and I couldn't blame them: it didn't seem to do much good. But I'd go in and laugh and joke with them, so they would give it a try and tell me what they'd like better.

I had visits while I was there from the doctor and from Molly as well, and they were pleased the patients were eating better. The doctor never said much to me, but I did just like to see him there. I'd go back to me bed of a night and dream he were stroking my arm, or our heads were touching like that first time, but Molly were quite strict, and very quick to get the ward nurses to learn how to make up the meals. So, it weren't long before I wasn't needed any more. Mebbe Molly wanted to see the back of me again, I dunno.

I didn't mind going back to Cook, though, and the main kitchen, even though I never saw my beautiful doctor again, and I didna' hear if my meals was doing any good for the lives of "my" patients. I could see Cook were pleased to see me back. I told her I never wanted to see another bowl of cream again, so she set me to peeling potatoes with Dorothy once more, who today was related to the Duchess of Devonshire, and knew a thing or two about cream and Jersey cows!

And I had time to think of all the things I'd learnt, and of how clever I'd been understanding all those new words and writing down the meals and weighing all the foods. Mebbe, one day, I'd cook in a proper kitchen, outside. But then it were safe in here: I always knew what to do, and I were never on my own.

XI

AGGIE WAS ALWAYS THERE WHEN I WENT BACK TO my bed, or the airing court, or to the day room. She never said owt, she never looked at me, or smiled. She were just there, beside me as soon as I arrived. I'd speak to her and mebbe she'd copy a word or two, or sing a verse of a hymn, and I'd think she must be content. I knew she were when she came to my bed o' nights, and so were I. She were still happiest drawing circles, though I tried to teach her some letters, but the only ones she learnt were ones with curls in them.

Liza still looked out for us both, but we didn't need her so much now. I still would read to her, and she'd help me with long words I didn't know.

"You're very clever, Liza," I said to her one day.

"Surely ye'll be making me out to be very grand, ye will."

"But you're strong, an' all."

"Now what gave you that idea?"

"'Cause you talk back to them as harry us."

"I've seen the worst they can do to us, and I'm not afraid. Besides, the voices chivvy me."

"Is that who you talk to, Liza, when you walk on your own… voices?"

"Ay, they're there all the time, have been since I were seventeen. Sure 'n some days I willn't listen, and some days they help, but mostly they chide me and torment me."

"Where do they come from?"

"Who knows. Mebbe the Devil? But whisht ye now. I don't talk of them, or they'll make me pay. And that's why I'll never get outta here, so best make the most of it."

She were stronger than even I had known.

"Read, child, read an' read an' read, and you'll learn a thing or two as'll help you… has me. Them as has power don't like us to, frightens them. But just think as where *Mrs Beeton* got you: making meals for patients."

"But what about Ruth, Liza? She's read books and she can talk posh but it has na' helped her."

"My heart surely breaks for Ruth. I feel her pain and her sadness like it were mine. She is sicker than all of us and I fear for her."

"Is she possessed?"

"Ay, by the melancholia. 'Tis the Devil itself drags her down to the Pit of Despair, into the miry clay, and she canna reach her learnin' to save her."

Some days later Ruth came back to us. Her hair was untidy and her pale skin grey. She had cuts and bruises around her wrists and I saw them on her ankles too when she undressed for bed. She looked more poorly still than she had before, and she moved not at all unless she were made to. Liza took to walking with her whenever she could, holding her up by her arm and talking softly to her. But we weren't there all the time and some mornings we left her in bed.

Some nights I'd go to her in her bed, and stroke her hair. Mostly she were just lying there, her eyes wide open.

"Tell me about the electric treatment, Ruth," I asked one night. "Did it help you?"

I thought I might get her to talk and that might make her feel better.

She turned and looked up at me. "No, Mary, it hasn't helped. I don't remember much of it. They put straps on me and gave me something to make me sleep and I ached all over after... that's all I know. They did it once every week and now I am just so tired."

"Will you see your baby on Sunday?"

"No, Mary, I've stopped seeing him. I cannot. He must not remember his mother like this. But I am too tired to care."

Aggie came over and sat on the bed and started stroking her hair as well, I don't know why. I didn't think Aggie could understand how other people felt. P'rhaps she just did it to copy me. Then she started singing "Dear Lord and Father of Mankind" and Ruth started crying, and I was glad 'cause I hoped the tears would help. And then she fell asleep and that was good as she never seemed to sleep. And I cried as well and went back to my own bed and Aggie followed me, and just for a little while we curled up together and I kissed her and I stroked her, and I stopped crying as my need for her grew until, all of a rush, I felt that heat and wetness and crampin' that always came from loving Aggie, and I knew from her sighin' that she felt it as well. And I wished that Ruth could feel it as I was sure it would make her feel good like it did me and Aggie. Then Aggie was gone, and the bed felt cold without her, and I was left to wonder again what it was she knew or cared about.

I would have done anything to make Ruth better, but I think Liza would have done even more. She never got cross with her and waited for her and walked with her, holding her so tenderly that she even made the nurses more patient.

97

But Liza and I had work to go to, and we didn't know what happened when we weren't there.

Then one morning Ruth would not get out of her bed. Liza and I had to leave her to go to our work.

Cook was grumpy. "Tha's late this mornin'. The Board of Visitors is here for lunch. I need some good pastry for apple pies, and steak and kidney prepared, and potatoes well pared for creaming. You can do that wi' Sally, but be quick."

Sally were one of the girls from the village "outside".

"Do ye know how to get the kidney ready?"

She shook her head, so I had to show her, then I did the pastry. I weren't going to let her do that, I were too good at it meself. But there was a lot to do, so I got Dorothy to do the potatoes, but I checked 'em after. And I were proud of what we sent in to them, and Matron came down later to thank us. So I was too busy to think on anything else till we were finished, then the nurses took us back to the day room.

It were very quiet in there. I couldna' see Liza or Ruth but Aggie was there, so we sat in a corner and Aggie drew circles and I read a book of poems out loud to her. I could ha' done with some help from Liza with some of the words, but we got by. We went to the dining hall for our tea and back to the day room and they were still not there so I began to worry about them.

Then it was late before we went to the ward for bed, and Ruth and Liza weren't there either. I asked one of the nurses.

"Never you mind," was all she'd say, but she looked agitated, like the nurses had when Liza had escaped, so I wondered if she'd gone again and taken Ruth with her.

I thought it best to sleep on it, but one of Liza's "ladies" came up to me and whispered, "Liza went to see her and never came back, y'know."

"Who?"

"Ruth, she never got up, so she went back to see her."

"How do you know?"

"Heard 'em talking. Said Liza was always a troublemaker."

"So where are they now?"

"Dunno."

There was nowt to do but wait till morning. But even then I could get no sense from anyone. So I went to the kitchens and asked Cook if she knew what had happened.

"I come in from the village in the morning, don't get to hear nowt, but I'll ask for thee."

I set to with veg to clean and onions to chop and it weren't till the end of the day that Cook took me to a storeroom and sat me down.

"I didna' know your friend Ruth; did she have the melancholia? Then that makes sense, for she killed hersel'."

I felt sick to my stomach. "How could she? She were weak as water."

"She hanged hersel' with sheets from her bed."

"How could they have let her?"

"She were asleep in bed when they left her."

"And what about Liza?"

"She went to see after her and found her. When the nurses came she were mad... attacked them, they were in fear of their lives. Had to take her off to the padd. Hush, don't ye cry, there's many as come and go in this place. Sometimes it's for the better."

"Never, never, never, Ruth had a baby, she were loved, and Liza loved her too. How could they lock *her* away?"

"Come, lass, dry your eyes. Ye're a good girl. Be strong. This'll not kill thee. It's sad but worse things happen, and we all keep going. Come back here tomorrow and we'll help thee start smiling again."

"I'll not be smilin' again."

"You will, as sure as eggs is eggs."

"But I might have helped her."

"And happen no-one could have helped her. Fret not, she's no more in pain. May the Good Lord bless her and keep her, and may she rest in peace."

"But Liza: what will happen to *her*?"

"Ye must wait and see. I canna tell."

So I went back to the day room once more and drew circles with Aggie till bedtime, when I cried myself to sleep and even Aggie couldn't comfort me. Then I waited and I waited, day after day, for Liza to come back.

XII

COOK DID HER BEST FOR ME. WHEN I ASKED her to find out, she said that Liza was on one of the back wards. They couldn't keep her quiet, kept keenin' so she did, and fighting when they shushed her, so she spent a lot of time locked in the padd, where she couldn't hurt herself or anyone else. Then she was moved out of the hospital and Cook didn't know where.

"I think that Miss Turner may have had summat to do with her move."

"Why, Cook?"

"I heard a whisper. That Molly and Liza didna' get by together."

"Mebbe, but I let her down, Cook."

"Of course ye didna, y' silly baby. She were a grown woman and a sick one if you ask me. There's many as live an' die in here: can't be takin' it to heart."

"I know. You know, I think Ruth would have ta'en her baby with her if she could. Liza couldn't bear that. I could never see that neither."

"Maybe you will one day. My fourth died of diphtheria. Slow it was. When you see someone sufferin' and you can do nowt, you want to take them where it can't hurt no more. For Ruth maybe life was just suffering."

"But her baby wasn't suffering..."

"How do you know? Who knows what Ruth saw for him in the future?"

"Why did they put me in here, Cook? I would have cared for *my* baby."

"You'd broke the rules, my dear. You were the temptress. You were Eve. You had to be locked away till men were safe from your temptation. It helped them to believe your wickedness was a form of madness."

"Was I wicked, Cook?"

"I wouldn't ha' said so, no more 'n the hen that squats for the cockerel, or the cats that wail in the night... 'tis nature's way. My firstborn was on his way before I married, no harm done, husband was a good man. Now get on with those spuds before I box your ears."

I felt better. She made me laugh.

Dorothy was laughing too. "When Adam delved and Eve span, who was then the gentleman?" and she spread her legs and threw her apron over her face.

Mostly we just cleaned the spuds but sometimes they had to be peeled and chopped. Today they were newly dug and young and earthy. The soil slipped off them, leaving them creamy and naked. They should've been boiled and eaten straight from the pot, but I knew that by the time they got to the plates they would be over-soft and sloppy, but what could you do when you were feeding so many?

I saved the best few to cook on their own for the doctors. We had some mint to chop to add to theirs as well.

I looked at my hands. The skin had wrinkled in the water

as I washed the 'taties. At the end of the day they were always red and sore. Cook would let me rub a little lard over them when I left the kitchens, and that helped.

"Dorothy, what was the best work you ever had?"

"Ask no questions and you'll be told no lies, madam. But I'll tell you a secret: I cooked for the Queen once."

I'd heard that one before. I still didn't know if t' were true or not.

"Queen Victoria, mind, not the Queen of Sheba. She were in t' workh'se."

"Who, Dorothy? Queen Victoria?"

"No, silly girl, the Queen of Sheba."

Talking with Dorothy could be very strange. Who was the Queen of Sheba anyway?

Dorothy wasn't from my ward. I only saw her in the kitchen, like most of the other women who worked in the kitchens. And the men who brought the veg and the meat from the farm. You could only get to see how many people there were in the hospital when they were all together in the dining hall or when the hospital put on "events". But even then that wasn't everyone. Them on the back wards didn't come for meals, and weren't allowed out for the "events".

The "events" were cricket matches, or a fair, or summat like that, and lots of people from "outside" would come into the hospital. Some of us could go along and watch, but we were watched ourselves all the time, and best behaved. It was the doctors and the nurses mainly who took part.

The nurses lived in the hospital and I never saw them leave it: not that I would have done anyway, I s'pose, but I think that was why it was exciting for them.

Then, from time to time there'd be "entertainments" for us, dances or a magic lantern show.

"Do you like the dances, Dorothy?"

"I do. Be better for a man or two, though. Favourite's the foxtrot. Shall I teach tha'?"

"I'll foxtrot you if you don't work a bit faster," Cook chivvied us.

We chopped and scraped and peeled in silence for a while.

"At the last dance we had music from a gramophone instead of someone playing the piano. That was good. And if you get to dance with Emily, she's real good. Most of the time it's just a shuffle, though."

"It's the Board of Visitors as asks for the "entertainments". When they meet they ask for a report on what's been organised." Cook had sat down beside us. It was rare to see her off her feet. "They like to think your time's well spent: work whenever possible, fresh air, exercise, mental stimulation and recreation. They think you're still in the workh'se, you can be 'reformed'. Have to show them what I feed y' as well. Then they complain of the cost.

"But you're in for a treat soon. I heard the Board of Visitors has said they should buy one of those cinematograph-thingys, so they can show films.

"You'll enjoy that. I enjoy a trip to the cinema. I may be just a Lancashire lass, but there's such a world out there as you wouldn't believe."

"Have you always worked here, Cook?"

"Nay, lass. I worked in the mill for many a year. Didn't have much edjecation but I was good at what I did, worked me way up to supervisor. Then met me husband, he was a supervisor too. We saved a bit o' money and took a shop on the edge of the town. Did well."

"So how did you learn to cook?"

"Just had to for me family. No different for three thousand. They took me here 'cause I said I could organise a kitchen and manage a body o' women. Done it in t' mill. And it were the war years: could find no others."

The door from the corridor swung open and Molly came in. She walked straight past me without a look. "Cook, I must speak with you about the diet for the tuberculosis patients on the Veranda ward." They walked off together where I couldn't hear them.

"Miss La-di-dah now she's Sister, and in the infirmary as well." Dorothy didn't really like the nurses, except when she thought they were someone else, or they'd been sent to her as some sort of heavenly messenger.

Molly came back and stopped in front of me; I thought she might speak to me, but she only half looked at me, then stared round the walls of the kitchen. But then she looked at me again. This time she held my gaze and I couldn't make out if she were angry with me or just weary. "Ah, Mary. One of the patients on the special diet has improved and is having fewer fits, so we're going to try it on another group of patients in the infirmary, but the nurses know what to do now so they won't need you." What had I done wrong?

She started to move away and then stopped again. "And I'm leaving, Mary, to go to the City hospital. I'm leaving this god forsaken place where nothing will ever change and no-one dares to put a foot out of place. Thank your lucky stars, Mary, that you come to work here in the kitchen. Cook is a free spirit. You'll get more sense out of her than everyone else put together in this lunatic place."

"Well, I go home o' nights." Cook had come up behind Molly. "I live in the real world out there. There's many in here as thinks the hospital's the real world, or even the whole world, and I don't mean just the patients. Got their clogs on backwards, they have. I know how to call a spade a spade. It helps."

Molly sighed. "I'm sure it does. So goodbye, Mary, take care of yourself." This time when she looked at me I thought she would cry, but then she turned away proper, her head shrunk into her shoulders, and walked slowly toward the door.

I took a deep breath. "Molly," I cried after her. "What happened to Liza?"

She turned slowly back toward me.

"It's not my place to tell you, Mary, but I suppose you were her friend. She was sent to another, more secure hospital, where she will be safe."

"Why, Molly, What hospital? What's 'more secure'?"

"Just another hospital. But I regret her going. She would have been a good ally in here. I never realised at the time but she knew things had to change, in here and outside, and she was right. I think I was almost as naïve as you when I arrived here, Mary, but I have changed. I am ashamed."

She was quiet for a long time. I waited for her to tell me more.

"But I do not have her courage. Goodbye, Mary." Then she walked to the door and out into the corridor, the lace tails from her cap flying all awry in the draught.

I didn't know what to say. I didn't understand what she was saying about Liza, and I was cross she wouldn't explain about the other hospital.

"Poor Liza. Why did they send her away? What will happen to her? Mayn't I see her again?"

"P'rhaps she'll come back again one day. Mebbe she's better off there, mebbe they'll be kinder there to 'er. You bide your time, and count your blessings."

"I suppose I *am* lucky, Cook. I suppose all of us as work in the hospital are lucky. It's good to work."

"There's plenty of you, mind. What came first: the chicken or the egg? The hospital couldn't work without tha', and tha' wouldn't work wi' out the hospital."

"But does it never change here, Cook? Molly said it wouldna' change. But there are lots of new young nurses now, come in place of the old ones. New ones with c'tificates and things. We have to call them Miss or Nurse, not by their Christian names anymore."

"But they still tell 'ee you're here for your own good, and they still turn you out into the airing courts, and lock you in at nights, and them's them and you's you. And when did you last make a decision for yourself, Mary?"

"It matters not how strait the gate, how charged with punishments the scroll. I am the master of my fate. I am the captain of my soul." A new voice in our talk made us turn.

"Dorothy, where did you learn these things?"

"Who knows, who knows."

I think Dorothy must have learnt bits of poetry by heart as a child, and still remembered them, but I was always surprised when she trotted 'em out and they were always so right for whatever we were talking about.

"I s'pose you're right, Cook. But I'm not sure I'd be any more a master of my fate 'outside', than I am in here. On the wireless they tell us there's no money, no food, and people's either on strike or unemployed." We'd just had a wireless set up in the day room. It was a great big wooden thing which made a lot of crackling noise when it was switched on, but sometimes you could tune it in well enough to hear the news, though the "ladies" in the day room tended to prefer it when we could find music on the dial. This, with the odd newspaper that found its way into the day room, gave us to know some little bits about the wider world "outside" to try to make sense of.

That world was changing, though, I could see that, and I didn't think I'd know it any more if I were "outside". I were always thanking God that I worked in the kitchen, as Cook and the girls from "outside" talked all around me about their lives, so I learnt more things from them. But *my* world were inside the hospital walls and here little changed. And I sought nowt more.

Every day I tried out my reading and writing, and I learnt my kitchen skills. Cook was a good teacher and was proud of my learnin'. She taught me everything I needed to know to keep all the patients and the staff fed, now over three thousand mouths. 'Course, this were pretty basic cookery, plain and filling food as always, making best use of what came from the farm; but along the way I learnt some butchery and some baking as well. But then Cook also had to cater for the doctors, and for visitors to the hospital, and for this she'd teach me more complicated things. I were a quick learner and good at changing what I'd learnt to fit what I'd got, something I'd done in my mind from my first days with Liza's *Mrs Beeton*. More and more I was trusted to suggest and put together special meals for these occasions. Then the visitors might come down to the kitchens to tell Cook they'd liked them, and I felt real proud of myself, though Cook never let on that it was my work. But she let me, from time to time, take a little pastry or a small tasting of something in aspic back for Aggie to try, though Aggie was very fussy about what she ate, and as often as not I ended up eating it mesel'.

Cook talked more to me as time passed. I liked to think she were more my friend. I had need o' a friend in here. One day she came and stood beside me as we cleaned and chopped some rhubarb, and told me more about her life. "I had four children, you know, Mary. The baby died but the other three were a strappin' lad and a couple o' lasses. The girls are wed now and I've five grandchildren."

"Where's your son now?"

"Ah, he were a warehouseman in the city. Volunteered at the beginning of t' war. Only sixteen he were, but lied about his age. Six foot tall he were, and strong, so they took him, no questions. Sent him to Heaton Park for training for months, then Salisbury Plain, then France. Hadn't been there two weeks when he was killed. I think that's what killed me husband."

"Were ye still working in the shop?"

"Aye, every hour God gave us. But we were doing well, well enough to buy us a little house just outside these walls. One of a terrace, two rooms downstairs and two up, with a little yard at t' back, and a tiny front garden opening on t' cobbles. It were grand… still is.

"But when our Jack never came back it broke his heart. He were older 'n me and he'd had rheumatic fever when he were a child, and his heart were weak. Dropped down dead in the shop one day. So that's why I gave up the shop and came here." She dabbed at her face with the hem of her apron.

"Look, I've a photo of Jack," and out of her apron she took a brownish faded picture of a young man in uniform. "Handsome, weren't he? Just like his father. That's the picture they put in the newspaper with his death notice. I always keep it with me, but I don't show it many." And she stowed it back in her apron pocket.

"He liked rhubarb, y' know. Funny the little things as you remember."

I had a sick feeling in my stomach. He were a part of her, like my baby were of me. He'd been ta'en away and never come back. My Peter were ta'en from me, but he were alive.

"There are many out there, like me, as would know your pain. The loss of a child, whenever…" Could she read my mind? "But such pain either breaks you or it makes ye stronger."

I might have asked her more but just then one of the nurses came into the kitchen.

"Cook, I must take Mary for her examination by the doctor."

I rinsed my fingers and she led me by the elbow into the corridor. I felt her hand move up my arm and then she pinched me hard. "Little miss la-di-dah, aren't we? Got Cook's ear, have we? No wonder we're getting fat."

I felt the tears pricking behind my eyes, but I knew if I cried she'd do it again. And I knew if I said owt she'd do worse, like tripping me up and standing on the hem of my skirt so I couldn't get up, "by an accident". So I just kept on walking. I knew if they really hurt us they had to leave the hospital, and when we bathed they had to check us for cuts and bruises, but it was more bother than it was worth to complain.

We carried on to the old anteroom and I waited there for my turn. These checks were now only once a year and quite quick, didn't undress you no more. I think they just had to show the Board of Visitors that we were all seen and were well, no "infestations" or consumption. They were really frightened of the TB. I had lost interest in them. I knew now there were no point in asking owt.

I *think* that they were annual inspections, but, to tell the truth, the months all merged into one another and it was difficult to keep track of the days of the week, let alone the years.

I was called in to see the doctor, a different one every time, though he were always at the same desk, and always writing in his ledger. I was weighed in my clothes and the nurse checked my hair for lice.

"How are you, Mary?" they always asked, but I don't think they really heard what you said. Then they put that listening thing on my chest, told me to breathe in and out, and that was it. I was free to go back to the kitchens again, taken, of course, by one of the nurses.

I didn't ask mesel' or them any more why I were here. It were just me an' Aggie now, and I counted Cook my friend.

One day there were a plague of flying ants, and ants without wings an' all, creepin' and crawlin' an flyin' in and out between the bricks that made the floor of one of the outside store rooms. Cook sent me with the vinegar to put down the cracks. We were just like those ants. I were one small ant in the great ants' nest that was the hospital: as long as we kept busy and out of sight we were all right, they didn't need the vinegar. Needn't try growing wings though.

The only things I had left of a different life were the doll, wooden body rubbed shiny from my bed clothes and joints rusted from my tears, having wet them so often, and Liza's *Mrs Beeton*. One day I'd give it back to her, I promised.

Part II

In the Shadow of the Bell Tower

I

1948

AGGIE'S SCREAMIN' HAS MADE ME HEAD ACHE, AND the echo of my feet and the voices in the corridor are making it worse. There's a group of people blocking my way back to the kitchens, and me and the nurse will have to squeeze past 'em. There's a tall gentleman with horn-rimmed glasses and a pink spotted bow tie (now that's a bit fancy for here!). He looks ever so lofty and commanding. He must be the new superintendent. And I can see two of the old Board of Visitors (not scurrying away as they usually do if you get too near 'em!). Who is that lady with them? I think I know her, though I'm not sure, perhaps she's the new deputy matron. The nurses have been full of chatter about the new Health Service, and of all the changes that are coming to us here, and, even if they don't tell us about 'em to our faces, they do gossip together, and we do earwig. We know there are going to be a lot of new people in charge. Though none of us have the measure of just how different things will be.

I think we are ready for some changes, though. We struggled through the war years. A lot of the staff, and most o' the doctors and the male nurses, left to join the Forces, so there were fewer of 'em, but not fewer patients. Then they turned some of the wards over to take the wounded, so we were crushed into an even smaller space. It were hard, and those of us with least problems found ourselves caring for t' others alongside the nurses. The wards and the corridors were sandbagged in case of bombs, though we were never hit, and we were all given gas masks. I had to take charge of my ward: my bit toward the "war effort", they said, keeping the hospital carrying on "as usual". If the air raid siren went off I had to make sure everyone had their gas masks and keep 'em calm, and when the nurses unlocked the ward door we had to head count 'em, and lead everyone down the corridors to the tunnels 'neath the hospital. They were hardly used now, but they joined up all the bits of the hospital that weren't joined up by the corridors. I never knew they were there before. They were very wide and dark and damp, though there were electric lighting, but it were quite poor; and they were tiled like the corridors above, so our footsteps and our voices echoed, and if anyone cried or screamed it were real scary. But we got used to going down there, and even Aggie would come without a murmur. Though I always put the old wooden doll in my apron, just in case (in case of what? I don't know). And I'd carry my *Mrs Beeton*, (or Liza's *Mrs Beeton*, I should say). And we'd sit down there on rush mats, and I'd get Aggie to sing hymns so we could all join in and make the time pass.

And then, of course, our numbers were swelled even further by new patients made ill by the fighting. Shell-shocked we used to call them when we saw them here after the last war. And they even sent patients from London hospitals on special trains to join us. So our ward was full to brimmin'.

And if I look round me I can see all the repairs that still need doing: there've been no men to do them. And the floors are not polished like they used to be, and the windows are smudged. How long will it take to get back to "normal"? Or mebbe we never will.

But the Chief Male Nurse catches my eye and takes me a bit way down the corridor. "Will you be cooking for us today, Mary? It's quite an important lunch, as you can see. Can I request the elderflower posset? I think our guests would enjoy it."

I smile. He's a nice man, though I don't see much of him. A bit bossy, mebbe, but he knows a good many of us by name, and he will stop and speak, and ask how we are as if he cares for the answer. And I know the elderflower posset is a favourite of his, so I am glad I got the lemons and the elderflowers ready yesterday.

The rest of the group have moved away, so I can't see them no more. So I go on to the kitchens, to the comfort of the steam and the rattle of the pans and the crockery, where Cook is struggling with a mountain of leeks.

"And have you settled madam Aggie down then?"

Cook and I have worked together for more years than I can number, and she is getting old now. She's well over sixty, but I think they kept her on as she's always been good at making scarce rations stretch. Over the years she has let me try out new recipes and cook them for the doctors and the visitors. Food were in short supply while the war was on: much of what the hospital farm produced was "requisitioned", but we didna' do too bad, and Cook wheedled the gardeners into growing things like borage and nasturtiums for me, things that grow like weeds but add colour and taste to simple food. The elderflower posset is one of my inventions, for elderflowers are easy got in May.

"Yes, thank you, Cook. I think she'll now go out to the airing courts. It were easier when we all had the same long skirts and aprons. Now we have a jumble of clothes to choose from, and Aggie gets upset if she don't recognise anything." I don't like the clothes we wear now, no more 'n she. They're supposed to be "modern", but they look more like "cast-offs", and it's difficult to find something to fit, let alone that looks pretty. The cloth is flimsy, and nowt has any shape. And we have to match them up with thick beige lisle stockings too. But then I have an apron to wear over them myself in the kitchen, so it doesn't really bother me, leastways not *too* much.

"Then don't dawdle. You have six soups to prepare."

"And three thousand dinners!" I laugh.

The kitchens run like clockwork; they have to. Cook still has a number of ladies from the wards working for her. She is good at knowing how best to use them. But more and more she has girls from "outside" to help. They don't last long though, they get frightened if our ladies talk to themselves or stare at them.

Mabel is from my ward. "How are you today?" I ask as I pass her, touching her shoulder on my way to find a sieve for my soup.

"No better for seeing you. We don't need you here," she replies, though she says it with a smile. But then she carries on her conversation with someone I cannot see. Mabel and I are good companions in the kitchen. She likes to sit in a quiet corner with a sack of potatoes, cleaning, peeling and chopping, watching the day go by, her hair cut short to her scalp ever since she had the "nits", and her back bent, with age, I s'pose. But she will let me help her, and sometimes she will help me, and then she likes to tell me a story, something she and her sister did when she was a child, or how she fell in love with the butcher's boy.

"Is it the new superintendent we're cooking for today, Cook?"

"Aye, and the new deputy matron. You can take the dishes in to 'em yourself, if you wish. Take a gander at 'em."

"If I sieve this soup, then, once more, it will be real smooth, and I'll warm the bowls so 'tisn't cold before they get it."

And I'm right. I did know the lady in the corridor. The new lady is Molly. Molly, who used to make us laugh with her jokes about spinster ladies, and who left and went away to become "a proper nurse". But she don't seem to recognise me, and I'm not surprised. Like Liza, she always said I were a child, and now I am grown. I have read and I have learnt, and I know more words now than you could believe. I read the newspapers, and I listen to the wireless. I followed the progress of the war as best I could, and the Charge found me an atlas so I could see where the countries were. And that Mr Churchill taught me a thing or two about words, as well, with his flowery speeches. So I write a journal now, and sometimes a little verse, to practise what I've learnt, and to play with all my beautiful new words. And I do it with Aggie as well, finding rhyming words that she will copy, and making them into rhythms that she will sing. Ah, there's two words to conjure with: rhyme and rhythm. I think it must be that h after the r, it makes them soft words to roll around tha' mouth.

And I've learnt to talk more proper (or should that be proper*ly*?) Don't sound quite right, though. I use right words now when I can: the girls from "outside" said they didna' understand my old-fashioned words and the way I said 'em. They say people don't talk like that now. They say the old "country" ways of speakin' are all dying out.

It were Liza I have to thank for my learnin'. What did she say? Ask a new question every day and find the answer. That's what I've done, and I'm proud of myself. And I am trusted: I know where I belong and what I have to do.

But it's some days before I see Molly again.

Molly was back to change things. She visited our ward at last late one afternoon. We were all in the day room, where at this time of the day we could sit and play card games or dice or read. The last superintendent had said we should have more books. I don't know where he got them, but at last they did arrive, many of them very old, battered and well-read, but so exciting. Jane Austen, George Eliot, Trollope, and some more modern novels as well: F Scott Fitzgerald, even John Steinbeck, and a dictionary, where I learnt a lot of my new words. He even got us the *Encyclopaedia Britannica*, the 1910 edition so it were a bit out of date, but I learnt a lot from that as well. And, best of all, I found tucked away among them, a little paper-backed copy of *Practical Camp Cookery for Guides and Guiders*. It were so much fun to read. Not that I learnt much from it. There weren't much that between them, my mother, Cook and Mrs Beeton hadn't taught me, but it reminded me of the days me and my brother spent with the charcoal burner, and I loved the idea of all those girls campin' outside together, lighting fires, and cooking in hay boxes. (Though I had no wish to do it myself; seemed the kind of thing only young people would do who had charge of nowt, and I had many as depended on me for their meals. I were proud of that.)

Aggie was sitting with me. She had now learnt to write her name. It pleased her a lot as it has curly circular letters in it: she was still taken with circles and anything that went round. She would spend hours with a pencil in her long thin fingers, drawing, as she was now. I loved her when she was quiet like this, I felt very close to her. She were very special.

"Look, Aggie, we can draw a daisy chain." And I drew a line of daisies and joined them up with "stalks". She took the pencil back from me and drew more daisies to make a circle, then she drew another circle of daisies inside the first. Then she sat back and smiled at her work and gave me back the pencil. She never seemed to get a mite older, her thick red curls still framing her long, pale face, and her eyes still far, far away, never holding mine, but she were calmer, and, in her own strange and silent, distant way, she shared her joys and her woes with me now. She would even let me touch her now, and put my arm around her, not just in bed, though she would still go stiff when I did it and turn her head away.

This were our quiet time, before we shuffled off to bed, a good time for Molly to see us. She blew into the room like the wind blowing through an open window, ruffling feathers and disturbing papers, "inspecting" patients, furniture, our books and games, with a word to the nurses about this, and a question about that. She came over to me and smiled. "So, you are still with us, Mary, and Aggie. And they tell me you do good work in the kitchen." She stood silently, staring at me, the smile fading from her lips, though it were never a warm smile; her eyes had never smiled anyways.

"Have you come back for good, ma'am?" I knew I couldn't call her Molly now. "I didna' think we would see you again."

"Yes, I believe I'm here to stay!" She bent toward me. Then, "Maybe there's work here for me to do. Maybe it was always my destiny." She talked so softly I could hardly hear her and I'm sure no-one else could. "Maybe because I hated it so much here I needed to come back, to conquer some demons. Perhaps there's unfinished business." For a few moments she looked deep into my eyes, and something in *her* eyes made me shiver. Or perhaps it was just the wind blowing in the still-open door. "Maybe you and I will always..." but then she turned away. "But we must have a longer talk some time." She said this more loudly, and not directly to owt in particular, as she straightened up and moved on.

I thought she were older and fatter than before, but then, so was I. But I had thought she would be more pleased to see me. I had thought we had memories that we might share and laugh at, and sad times we might remember an' all. I felt empty, disappointed, I suppose; I remembered what a child I had been when she came, and how I had missed my mother then, and how Molly had seemed to bring life into our dreary days. But mebbe I didn't want to think back to that time either; it pained me too much. And it was over. This was my life now, here with Aggie, and working in the kitchens.

Molly and her nurses came to the end of their walk around the day room and blew out the door again. It was time for bed. The sinking sun was still shining through the high windows of the ward as we undressed. It was so low you couldna' look out through the glass or it dazzled tha', and it sent long, long shadows across the floor, till it hid behind the bell tower and the sky turned pink around it. We, Liza's "ladies", undressed quickly, as we always did: we had no time for modesty. The key turned in the lock on the ward door, the scrape and clang we were used to, and several dozen women settled down to cough and grumble and dream the night away, as Aggie slipped into my bed. The sheets were rough and cold, but Aggie was warm and soft beside me and I felt safe. I didn't need owt else. I didn't need Molly.

II

AFTER HER FIRST COLDNESS, MOLLY SEEMED to have taken to me. She oft searched me out. Usually it was to ask if I would cook a certain dish for a visitor, or give her a recipe for summat, but always she was distant, and often I felt she stopped, as if there were something else she wanted to say. Today she has come to the kitchens to talk to Cook, but she stands by my table.

"Mary, have you ever been outside these walls since you arrived?"

"No, ma'am."

"Do you not wish to?"

"No, ma'am, not now." There was a time, when my baby were just born, and my mother were alive, when I would have given anything to have left this place. I hated it, and I hated the people who had brought me here. But my baby will be a grown lad now, and my mother is dead, so what is there for me out there? The people I care about are here, and I like my job in the kitchens. I would be frightened crossing the road out there, and people would stare at me. I am just another "lunatic".

"I am happy here."

"We could find you work outside the hospital, cooking, perhaps."

"No, thank you, ma'am."

She shrugs her shoulders and wanders away.

Then she comes back, another day and another day, with the same questions. I wish she wouldn't.

One day she invites me to her office. "Come, Mary, have a cup of tea with me." I sit on the edge of the easy chair she points to. Her office is quite small when you're used to the wards and the kitchens, but the ceiling's high and there are lots of pictures on the walls. I can't see them well, but mostly they seem to be photographs of the hospital before the war, nurses in their uniforms, and people I don't recognise. But there is one picture full of colour: a painting, I think, of flowers in a vase, with a bowl of shiny fruit beside it on a table and a curtain behind. I think it must be clever to paint like that. The picture is on the wall behind a great desk covered in papers and books. I think it would make me smile having a painting to look at every day like that, like the flowers we always used to have on the ward table when I first arrived in the asylum. We don't have those any more.

Molly makes a pot of tea and puts it on the table in front of me. Then she fetches two cups and sugar and milk, and sits in the chair opposite. "Now, Mary, surely you would like to earn some money for yourself. You could buy yourself some clothes of your own."

"Why would I want to do that? I wear an apron all day in the kitchen. Mebbe if we *all* had our own clothes…"

"But would you not like some really nice clothes? New clothes in nice fabrics, with silk stockings and pretty shoes. We could find you a job outside the hospital. You could continue to live in the hospital, at least to start with. Then you might like to look after yourself, have a place of your own. You could

124

go to bed when you wanted, and get up when you wanted. Eat what you liked, go to the cinema…"

It's like she is pleading with me, but she is vexing me and making me very anxious. "Molly," I feel I can use her name in this little room. "I amn't stupid, I know the world has moved on. We have a better wireless now in the day room, and we can listen to it in the afternoons before we go to bed. And newspapers get left us, and the *Woman's Weekly* still comes from time to time. Clothes are different, Molly, and there are cars on the roads. And what would I do with the money? I don't even understand the pennies now, nor what things cost. I wouldn't know how to pay for things."

When I think about it I can feel my heart beating real fast, and I can't breathe.

"Anyway, I know ladies cook and clean for themselves now, so what would I do? And sometimes we listen to *Music While You Work* on the wireless in the kitchens; lots of girls work all day in factories or offices now. They listen to this music all day, and then go home to their beds in rented rooms, so what's so different about my life?

"And I am ignorant. I know that. I have learnt a lot and I read and I can write, but the world I learn about is a dream. I have no schooling. Out there I would be a laughing stock."

"No, Mary, you're an intelligent woman. There aren't many that I would speak to like this in here. You have great potential. You have much to offer the world outside, and it has much to offer someone with your enquiring mind. Perhaps you should never have been in here at all, but we can't go back; we must look to the future."

I sip my tea. It has a strange flowery smell to it, not like the strong stewed brew we drink with our breakfast. She offers me a biscuit. "These are my favourite, Mary. Garibaldi biscuits. My nieces call them 'squashed fly' biscuits."

She sighs. "Mary, I really want to get you out of this place."

"Why?" What right has she got...

"I don't know, Mary, perhaps I owe it to you."

That doesna' make sense, and she says it so softly I can hardly hear. But then she stands up suddenly, all stiff and starchy again. "We cannot reverse things that have happened in the past but we can make sure girls like you aren't locked up now. And those that have been, we should return them to their families."

"Most of 'em wouldn't want to go; this is their home now. And I have no family mesel' anymore."

"No, Mary. I should remember, you're just another 'lunatic', that's what we would have said, isn't it? When you were first here." She's lost patience with me. "Why am I hitting my head against a brick wall? You've been here too long.

"Have another biscuit, and let's talk of something else."

She sits down again and pushes her hair back from her forehead. It's shorter now and not so tightly curled and pinned, but it's still as corn-coloured as ever. She shouldn't eat so many biscuits, though.

"Who painted that picture, Molly?"

"My brother. My dear sweet brother. He's really quite talented." Her face has gone red but she's calmer again. "It's a copy of a picture by a much more famous French artist. He taught our nieces to paint (my brother, I mean, not Cézanne)." She manages a half smile. "He was very patient. He never married, though, you know. He's a publisher." She's quiet for a minute or two, then, "But I have another idea, Mary.

"All the doctors and the senior staff, and our visitors as well, love your cooking. We have many compliments. And people often say that the dishes are unusual, or they've never tasted such combinations of flavours before. Cook used to say you had a gift, imagination that could turn an old recipe into something new and wonderful.

"What if you were to write down your inventions and we put them together in a book? We could see if my brother would publish it. I think lots of people would buy it. As you said, most women are cooking for themselves now and they're on the lookout for cheap, simple and quick recipes but with something special about them. And you use ingredients they could grow in a back garden or on an allotment, or even on a windowsill."

She's getting quite excited, but so am I. Well, a bit anyway. She jumps up and rifles through the stuff on her desk.

"Here you are, Mary, a notebook, and let me find you some pencils. Ah, here. Take them. What do you think? A good idea?"

I'm not sure what to say. I have jotted down recipes and ideas for recipes from time to time. I used to make lists of ingredients and play around with them when I was first practising my reading and writing. Then I used to write on the old butcher's block paper.

"I could try."

"Excellent. We have a plan. Now I must get on with my work. Come back and have tea with me again when you have something to show me." Then she takes my cup, opens the door and bustles me out of the room. I am left feeling a bit lost in the corridor outside, but I soon gather my wits and wander off toward the day room.

I think long and hard about her idea. I would like to see my recipes written down, and even better, in a little book like that old copy of *Mrs Beeton* of Liza's. I go to bed still thinking, but wake in the night.

I climb out of the bed and sink onto the floor beside it. It is after dawn, but the morning bell has not yet been rung. Soon I must get dressed, but as I got out of bed my legs gave way beneath me. The floor is cold. I cannot stop the tears coming, and the pins and needles in my chest. I am holding my baby again, his fingers wrapped around my little finger. I can smell him, I can feel him, but then he's gone again. All I have is the doll, wood and wire. I try not to remember, remembering hurts like a real pain, like a knife deep in my belly, but Molly forcing me think of "outside" makes it all come back. And all her talk of family… that were cruel. Nothing can bring my baby back, and leaving here won't help. I am so alone, so lonely; I would be even more alone out there. If I did find him now he wouldn't want me. Why should he? But he was so beautiful, so perfect. And I made him; he was mine.

I have no Liza now to chide me and make me face the day, but I must see to Aggie, so I slide my back up the polished tiles of the wall until my legs will hold me again, and I take a deep breath, as the morning bell rings, the key turns in the lock, and the nurses come through the door for their day shift. I will not let them see me cry, I will not.

III

IF MOLLY WANTS TO UNSETTLE ME, SHE'S NOT the only one, and neither am I the only one to be unsettled. I think the new superintendent has some fresh ideas. The nurses are very jumpy. They huddle together in corners. We hear them talking to each other. "There is another meeting about this 'open doors' policy. Will you be going?" a tall young woman pushing dark curls under her nurse's cap asks another over our heads in the day room.

"Shall we have the wireless on?" she says vaguely to no-one in particular as she tidies the books scattered on the table.

Then she turns back to her companion, who yawns as she replies, "I don't know. I may be on duty. Matron keeps saying we must remember this is a hospital now, not a prison, and not an asylum, but you know who'd be blamed if any of them escaped."

Are we invisible, or deaf? I want to slap them.

"I don't think they should have made the mental hospitals part of the new National Health Service. They need a different kind of management."

"Matron says we're here to care for patients, though, just like any other hospital."

"Mad, bad, or sick, are they?"

"Matron says they are all patients, and therefore here for treatment, not custody."

"I still say it'll make our job twice as difficult if they're allowed to wander. And what treatment would you offer someone like Mary, or Aggie for that matter?"

As usual they walk away, still talking, as if we weren't there.

But things do change. No-one talks to *us* about it, but suddenly the ward doors *are* unlocked, and left unlocked, at least during the day, and we are told we can go anywhere at any time, except outside the hospital grounds. And do we escape? Well, why should we? For most of us this is our home. But, though I've had quite a lot of freedom to come and go between the kitchens and the farm for a while, I really like being able to choose myself when I go, and then I'll wander down to the big field past the banks of rosebay willowherb, down to where they keep the chickens and the geese. The geese, the silly things, come running over to me to be fed, wobbling from side to side, their long necks reaching out as if they're in a race, and often I'll find something to bring them from the kitchens, or windfall apples from the orchard, and they snatch them from my fingers, while the chickens cluck round my feet.

And when the sun shines Aggie and I can find a patch of grass to sit on, and make daisy chains, or lie and watch the clouds moving who knows where through the vast blue of the sky above.

"Do you see the shapes in the clouds, Aggie? Hey diddle diddle, can you see the dish running away with the spoon?"

And she'll not reply, or she'll sing the rhyme, or watch the clouds through her fingers, lacing them together to make peep-holes of different shapes and sizes.

A few of the patients do take work outside the hospital, but they are mainly men and not from our ward, and we only know that because Cook tells us. She also tells us that it has been agreed that we should have some payment for our work inside the hospital, and we can ask for this money if we want to go out to the village "outside" to spend it. Mostly the money buys cigarettes, and quickly "cigs" are used like money in here.

Not that people didn't smoke before, but mostly it was under the eye of the nurses, and cigs were doled out as bribes or rewards. Now cigs can be got anywhere and the men can be seen sneaking a smoke away from the wards and away from supervision. Even some of the ladies do it. I tried it once, but I didna' like it, made me feel dizzy.

Now when I leave the ward I meet people from other wards in the corridors or out in the grounds, women and men. To be truthful they rarely speak to me, and I have no need of their chatter. T' other day, though, I saw one of the ladies from our ward coming up from the orchard, where the grass has been left to grow. She were kissing this lad from one of the men's wards and touching the private parts of his body and I were shocked; but then I suppose we're all used to having no privacy, sharing our bodies and all our private functions on the ward. And if she wants to fuck him why shouldn't she? Better 'n peeing in the airing courts in front of everyone like as some used to. Many of us have no seen men for a very long time, and have lost respect for our own selves.

Next, though, we are all "invited" to a meeting. It is held in the day room on the ward and most of our nurses are there, as well as Molly, the Matron, and the Superintendent. One or two of the young doctors are there as well. And, of course, we, the "patients", are there; we do as we are told. We sit on chairs in a circle. It's a large circle in a large room, and it feels strange as the rest of the furniture has been pushed up to the walls. It's also cold, as the fire hasn't been lit, but there is plenty of light streaming through the windows. We're not used to sitting together like this, and I can see some of the ladies itching to get up and walk around.

The Superintendent says he's pleased to see us all here. He tells us that there are to be meetings, once a week, every week, here on the ward. We do not have to attend but we all can if we want.

"The purpose of the meetings is to share ideas about how we feel the ward is running. We can think about how we work together, and how we can help each other." He smiles. I wince!

"Who will chair the meetings?" asks one of the doctors.

"No-one, and every person will be equal and free to say whatever they want." The young doctor shrugs but says no more.

There is a long pause.

Molly is sitting forward on her chair, but most of the nurses are leaning back, as if they're not really part of the goings-on, with their arms folded, and frowns on their faces. Most of our ladies are fidgeting, or rocking back and forth on their chairs, or looking out' window.

"The meetings will last an hour and no longer, so those of you who have work to do will not miss much."

A little voice inside me wants to ask if anyone will bother to listen to us, the patients, if we speak, but my heart thumps inside my chest so hard I daren't.

"These will be private meetings. Nobody from outside the ward will come, and we will respect each other and listen to each other. We won't gossip about what's been discussed with anyone outside this room. This is a step on the way to the hospital becoming a therapeutic community." He smiles at Molly and I think they must have hatched these ideas together: no-one else seems pleased. Matron sighs, takes her glasses off and rubs her eyes with her hand.

"If we can express what is bothering us we are halfway to understanding ourselves, and well on the road, with the help of others, to addressing our problems. A therapeutic community heals itself."

That makes little sense to me, but I take a deep breath. I shall say what's been bothering me for a long time. "So can we have our own clothes, please? I think that would help us." I can't say anything more as my heart is beating so fast and my hands are trembling, and my stomach feels as if it's jumped into the back of my throat. I don't like speaking with everyone watching and listening.

But that has floored 'em!

"The laundry couldn't cope with that, Mary," chip in several voices at once. "How would the clothes be sorted?" "Everything would have to be labelled." My goodness, you'd think I'd asked for silver spoons in the dining room; they've nearly jumped out of their seats!

Ah, well, I tried. At least it woke 'em up. But I mean it. How can we be anything more than "just lunatics" if we have no identity? I looked that up in the dictionary once, identity: something to do with the fact of being who or what a person is. If our clothes identify us, but we don't have our own clothes, how can we ever be more than "just lunatics"?

The room is quiet again. There seems to be nothing more anyone wants to say, so the Superintendent ends the meeting and we all wander back to what we were doing before. I take Aggie back to the airing courts before I return to the kitchens.

"Will they really listen to us if we tell them what'll make our lives easier, Cook?"

"Who knows. Seems a daft idea to me. Wastin' time."

"What do *we* know about how to organise a hospital?"

"It's your home, though. Maybe there are things you could

change. But it's no bother to me now, Mary, I'm old and my bones ache, and I'm leaving at last."

"Why, oh dear, what'll happen without you? Oh my goodness."

"Never fret, Mary. There's a grand new chef coming to take my place. I've told him of you, and the other ladies as well, of course. He'll bring some new ideas with him, I expect, but that'll be good. And I shall have a little pension and go and live with my daughter, and then I can rest these old bones and cook nothing but toast and a brew for the rest of my days."

"But you're my friend, I shall miss you. Will you come back and see us?"

"Perchance, but you must visit me: Miss Turner tells me she wants you to leave the hospital. My daughter would be happy to see you."

So Molly has been talking to other people about me. "Cook, how can I ever be part of that world outside!"

"Silly woman. Would you stay here for ever? What's wrong wi' ye?"

"They called me a moral defective. I had a baby."

"Ay, I knows that, but you were no more 'n a baby yourself, and 'tis not unheard of in this day and age for a lass to have a bastard child, but they don't lock you up for it now."

"Would they take your baby from you now, though?"

"No, but most girls would still give 'em up, for adoption, if they didna' have a 'usband."

"And never see them again. So things don't change that much."

"Nope, but that don't mean tha' canst not make tha' way int' world, so finish those carrots for me, and remember: I shall expect tha' visit. There'll be nobbut else to tell me the hospital gossip."

IV

SOMETIMES THE TIME PASSED VERY SLOWLY in the hospital, and sometimes the years seemed to flash by. Soon we were used to "open doors", and the weekly meetings. Molly stopped mithering me about going "outside", but she were more busy with other things, as she took to being matron when the old matron retired. I liked the new man in the kitchen. He were very tall and had silver hair and a very deep voice. He and Molly both reminded me about writing down my recipes, so I did that in my free time in the afternoons in the day room. Molly even suggested I come and do it in her office and learn how to use the typewriter there, but that would have meant leaving Aggie on her own, and I didn't want to do that, well, not reg'lar anyways.

We still didna' have our own clothes, even though I'd said so many times at the meetings that we could wash them ourselves, and store them on the ward if we had our own cupboards or shelves. Now that we could walk round the hospital grounds as we wished it made me sad to see the men looking like lost souls, shuffling along in suits with the sleeves too long or too short, and shoes with no laces, and the ladies with dresses that didn't fit 'em, with belts to tie them up as didn't match, and stockings that wrinkled round their ankles. If we had our own clothes we could choose things that fitted, and that we looked nice in. For sure we looked more like "lunatics" now than we ever did in our skirts and aprons.

The meetings did have some uses, though. It helped us to know each other a little better. Now I understood it was her sister that Mabel talked to all the time. They always slept in the same bed together, and her sister died in that bed beside her when Mabel was twelve. She'd been with her ever since.

And Doris, when she leant over to me in the meetings, grabbed my wrist and hissed to me to stop watching her, that was her "paranoia". She didna' mean ill by it.

But the meetings were still only held on our wards and not the back wards, though I thought as how Molly wanted to change that, for she brought nurses from there to our meetings, and I could see her sweet-talkin' 'em.

There were new young doctors in training in the hospital now, and medical students, and trainee nurses in smart new cotton uniforms with short skirts, but they were not allowed to come to the meetings unless we invited them. No-one was allowed to come unless they were a patient or worked regularly on the ward, unless we invited them. But Molly would wheedle her nurses in. We had been asked if we would allow Sister Matthews from Ward 14, one of the back wards, to attend, and, of course, we said yes. We knew Molly wouldna' let us say no, and anyway I think we were curious about this woman and what she might say. It were a game: we watched the visitors to see how much they squirmed in their seats, and if they said summat we waited for the doctors or the nurses to answer and then we all pitched in. It were like a dog fight of words!

So here she is today.

"Thank you for inviting me," she says as she introduces herself, but she doesn't look happy to be here.

She sits upright in her chair with her back stiff and straight and her arms folded across her tightly buttoned chest, as a few more people shuffle in.

One of the doctors is looking at his notes.

Doris is unpicking the hem of her dress. I think there must be a loose thread.

The chairs are hard. I can't decide whether 'tis more comfortable sitting straight with my knees together and my ankles together, or with my legs crossed. I try one then t' other. Does it make any difference?

Someone coughs.

Flecks of dust dance in the shafts of light shining through the high windows.

We wait for someone to say summat. Usually 'tis one of the nurses as starts us off, about something as has happened on the ward.

"We have decided to close the ward after breakfast each day while it is cleaned." The Ward Sister (used to be the Charge) begins. "You won't be able to return till the afternoon. This will allow the cleaners to do their work unhindered. The day room will still be accessible."

"We used to clean the wards and make our own beds before! And the nurses used to help!"

"Mary, you're not here to do menial tasks like that, and we're not here to be skivvies, or to spend our time supervising bed-making and sweeping."

"Well then, can we not be rid of the commodes on the

ward at night? That would help the cleaners, and mebbe the ward wouldn't smell so bad."

"What would you do without them?"

"If the bathrooms and lavatories were unlocked at night we could use them."

There is a look of horror on the Ward Sister's face. "That could be dangerous."

The doctor doesn't even look up from his notes. "They're already free to escape or hang themselves during the day now. Why not at night?" I shiver. I remember Ruth. Locked doors didn't stop her.

"It seems a reasonable request to me." Molly is smiling. "Why don't we give it a try and see how it's working next week." I see some of the other nurses welcome this as well. But it won't happen on Ward 14. Our visitor's arms are crossed even more tightly across her chest!

"The hospital has appointed a new occupational therapist. He will be setting up some arts and crafts sessions for some of you and some simple paid work if you wish it."

"Is that better 'occupation' than cleaning the wards then?"

"Many of you have nothing to do all day."

"Many of us are used to proper work."

"Took pride in cleaning the ward, we did."

"It were our home."

"See what he has to offer. You may like it."

"Putting the tops on squeegee bottles, huh!"

"Can't take no pride in that, and just for pennies."

"He'll have more creative things for you to do as well."

We fall silent again. These seats seem to get harder.

The doctor raises his head from his notes, and, looking straight at Doris, he asks why she keeps telling everyone she wants to kill him.

I try not to giggle. I would have thought that was plain

simple. He doesn't really like us. We're not "interesting" enough. Doris doesn't like the way he looks down his nose at her, and neither do the rest of us, but the rest of us aren't brave enough to say owt. Doris takes it to heart though.

"Tha's not so high and mighty. Tha may think tha' be."

"But what do those words really mean?"

There follows a useless "to and fro" about the meaning of what we say to each other, while Doris mutters under her breath, "I *will* kill him!"

And so it goes on, until the meeting ends.

Molly calls me over. "This is Sister Matthews, Mary. Sister, there is someone on your ward I'd like Mary to meet. I think she will know her."

"She may come if she wishes, but the ward is very understaffed, Matron, as I have told you before."

"I know, Sister, but maybe there are other things we could do that would make your life easier."

"I cannot supervise a wardful of women with the number of staff I am allocated. It is impossible."

We walk together to Ward 14. Sister leads the way at a brisk pace. She unlocks the heavy door and stands back for us to enter as if she is a magician opening a black box. And black it is. I am taken aback by what I see. It is a long time since I've been on one of the back wards. I was last there when I helped the young doctor with his diet for the patients who were taken with the fits. But that ward was part of the infirmary and this ward is very different. It seems to be divided by an invisible barrier into two areas. At the near end the patients are free to walk around, though there is little for them to do, but at the far end the ladies are sat, unmoving, staring at the floor, or at their hands, or out the high windows. They are sat on benches pinned behind a large table. And the ward smells of urine and worse. "Those are my 'wet and dirties', Matron. This is the only way I can meet their needs. They need individual supervision. They are happy to sit where they are told, and this way I can confine the tasks they set my nurses."

"Perhaps if you gave them more freedom, more ability to choose…"

"That's been tried. Just makes more work for us. Quite a few of them are on the new medicine, the Largactyl. That's made things easier. It calms them down, but it can make them more unsteady on their feet and more likely to be incontinent."

We move down the ward and I notice that the washing areas open off the ward in the same way as ours do, but, glancing through the open door, I see that there are no doors inside on any of the bathrooms or the lavatories.

Molly takes me over towards the seated ladies, leans over, and takes one of their hands. A shock of grey, dishevelled hair covers the face, chin dropped upon her chest. At the touch the head slowly lifts, and two eyes gaze blankly at Molly's face, and I feel sick. It is Liza. Does she recognise me? I think so. Her eyes soften as they turn to me. "I thought you had gone to another hospital, Liza."

"She did," Molly says gently, "but they sent her back here when they felt she was no longer a danger to herself or anyone else. So how are you today, my dear?"

The eyes fill with tears, and I kneel beside her to see better into her face, but she says nothing.

"Mary will come every day and take you out of the ward for a short walk till you start to feel better. Sister, that will be all right with you? It'll be a small contribution towards easing your staffing problems. Mary, you can come in the afternoons after you've finished in the kitchens."

I take both of Liza's hands in mine and squeeze them tight. "I will be back tomorrow, I promise."

I am late now for the kitchens, so we hurry away. Molly's face is set. She looks angry and I wonder that her new ideas haven't reached Ward 14. Before I leave her, though, she stops. "If you are going to help with Liza you need to know a bit more about what has happened to her.

"She was sent to Broadmoor Hospital, because that was where they sent the 'criminally insane', the ones who would have otherwise gone to prison. She became extremely disturbed and was threatening to kill the nurses here after she witnessed that young woman's hanging, and it was felt it would be safer there." She means Ruth, not "that young woman"! And she doesn't need to be so impatient with me; *she* took me to Ward 14, I didn't ask to go.

"Liza has an illness we now call schizophrenia and she has good times and bad times. Recently she has been bad again and has started treatment with Largactyl, our so-called new miracle drug. But she can have very good times, as she did when we first knew her. Liza had probably been ill for some time before she first came to the asylum. She smothered her own baby. And she attacked her husband with a knife, though that may well have been provoked. It was her husband had her committed, though she would have been tried and sentenced for killing her baby in any case. All this is public knowledge, though we kept it from the other patients. So I'm not breaching her confidence. Broadmoor has taken many women who have killed their own babies in the past, but it's changing. It's come under the new NHS, like all of us. And that's when they sent her back here.

"Liza sometimes believes some very strange things, and it can be difficult to know whether what she tells you is true or the deception of her troubled mind. If you are to help her you need to understand that her mind is very confused.

"Broadmoor was good for her, I think. I don't think we're helping her much here now, though, but I'm sure we can do better. The new treatments are good, and they say the Largactyl helps to suppress the voices that patients like Liza hear. I worry, though, that it makes them too sleepy so it knocks the fight out of them, and then they can't do anything to deal with the voices themselves. But, no doubt we will learn to use these new treatments better in time.

"I think Liza has come to some sort of terms with her voices before, and I know she is an intelligent woman. Maybe you can help her to regain her self-respect so she can cope with life again."

"But you never did like her, Molly, did you?" I will not let her talk to me like this, as if I am here just to do her bidding, as if she cares, as if she knows it all, as if she has all the power.

"You couldna' bear her keening, so they said. They said it was you sent her to Broadmoor."

"No, I admit that I didn't care for her. She was a thorn in my side, with her socialist principles, her women's rights, her championing of the underdog. She challenged so many things I held dear. But I didn't have the authority then to send her away. Though I might have done if I could. But I came to miss her… even admire her. I have learnt so much, Mary, since those early days. I have so many regrets."

She has caught her breath again after the dash from Ward 14. And the look on her face has softened.

I don't know what to say. What regrets can she have? She's done all right for herself! And she's giving me nursing duties as well as kitchen duties now! What do I know about these fancy names and fancy new treatments?

"So, will you help, Mary?"

"Well, I can but try," I manage.

My head is still reeling from the shock of seeing Liza again, and from what Molly has told me about her. And I'm still angry with Molly. But I'd like to help Liza, not for Molly's sake, or for Sister Matthews, or for anyone else. Maybe I can get my old friend back. She *was* my friend, though I wonder now if I ever knew her properly. But I could talk to her, even though she called me a child. I have no-one now I can share my thoughts with, except Aggie. Perhaps if I had a friend I could face leaving the hospital more easily. But was I *her* friend? She kept those secrets to herself. But mebbe she had to. Come back, Liza, and we can be strong together again. Please come back to me.

V

I HAVE NOW BEEN TAKING LIZA FOR WALKS IN THE hospital grounds every day for several weeks. She still says very little, but she looks better. I think the medicine they give her makes her quite sleepy and unsteady on her feet. But she's not wet anymore and she smells better, thank goodness. One day we found a bench and sat on it and I brushed her hair and tied it back the way she used to have it. She seemed to like that. Of course, I talk all the time, usually about the early times when we were all together, and sometimes that makes her smile. I can't understand how she can have changed so much. And I am really having trouble thinking about what Molly told me. I suppose it makes sense of why Liza would never let me talk of my baby, but what of all the other things she told us?

Today I've brought Aggie along. She is trailing behind us. She has taken no notice of Liza at all. I have linked arms with Liza. If I didn't we would never get anywhere. Aggie has started singing, just softly to begin with, but now I can pick out the tune. It's "Dear Lord and Father of Mankind". We used to sing that when we bathed. I join in.

"Breathe through the heats of our desire
thy coolness and thy balm,"
then Liza's voice quavers;
"let sense be dumb, let flesh retire;
speak through the earthquake, wind and fire."
We stop, and, just as it used to, Aggie's sweet, sweet, high
voice rings out alone:
"O still, small voice of calm;
O still, small voice of calm."
Liza smiles. "Sure, and those were good times." It is good
to hear her speak. And Aggie smiles to herself as well. I'm sure
she remembers and this is her way of telling us that.
We continue walking.
"We missed you when you went away."
"They took me. I told them they had killed Ruth. She told
me they were feeding her poisons."
"Ruth didn't care to eat. She weren't being poisoned."
Silence as we walk further. Aggie is singing again, but very
softly.
"I still have your *Mrs Beeton*, Liza. Do you want it back?"
"Ruth is here, you know. They tell me I must watch
for her. She was buried in the churchyard. But I see her.
She comes to the ward. She asks me where her baby is."
Liza's eyes open wide and she stares at me. Drawing back
from me she pulls her arm from mine. She is shaking and
she looks terrified. "No, 'tis your baby that is lost. Find the
pillow. Take it away. They said I had to do it. It can surely
be undone."
She turns and starts to run, but she is easy to catch. I hold
her in my arms. She is sobbing and trying to push me away.
Aggie is marching round and round us, her hands over her
ears, singing louder and louder. I want to scream, and I want
to hit Liza. I want to shake her. I want to hurt her. I want her

to be the person I knew before. How could she kill her own baby? No wonder she understood Ruth so well.

And then she starts screaming and a couple of male nurses appear from nowhere. "Which ward, love?"

"Fourteen," and I turn around and walk away. I feel ashamed. I am guilty. I have abandoned her. But no, you never really cared, Liza, no-one cared. You never held *me* when my baby was gone. You were kind and sensible, and did what was right, but you never really, really cared. No-one has ever really understood. I am alone and I hate you for needing me. I can't help you. Only Aggie ever holds me, and what does she understand? Who knows?

I return to the ward and my bed, and Aggie follows. I find my stack of papers and my notebook, and take them to the day room to work on, but the words swim before my eyes… flour, water, salt and vinegar: pastry for a bitter pie, filled with anger and regret, but nothing *can* be undone.

"Oh, Aggie, what have we done? Why are we here? What happened to Ruth? Stay here, I have to find out. But I will be back, my love."

I leave the papers, I leave the day room, I leave Aggie. I walk the long corridors, my footsteps echoing as I go. I take the shortest cut and cross the grass to the administration block. I go up to Molly's door. "I want to know what happened to Ruth, I want to find her grave, and my mother's. I'll leave the hospital to find them. I need to know where they are, and I need to touch them. Molly, ma'am, Matron, whoever you are, whoever you think you are, you must do this for me. You owe it me."

She is not alone. I think it's her brother, but he is gone before I can take him in. He seems to fade away through the door as I burst in. Molly looks upset, and suddenly I feel foolish and guilty as well as angry.

"Sit down, Mary, and calm down. Now I was waiting for you to ask me. I thought one day you would want to know. Patients who die in the hospital or who passed away in the past in the workhouse have always been buried in St Peter's churchyard, unless their families have claimed them and they can afford to pay for a funeral and a burial. They have generally been buried six to a grave, in unconsecrated ground in a corner of the churchyard, and usually the graves have been unmarked, or marked with a cheap stone or wooden marker, the kind of thing that will have deteriorated by now. We are trying to change that, but it's difficult. No-one laid claim to your mother's body when she died in the workhouse, but we know whereabouts she is buried. I can take you there."

It's as if she has prepared this speech.

"I don't think Ruth's family could afford to pay for her burial, and anyway she committed suicide, and that's still a crime, even now, though thank goodness I think the law is becoming a little more compassionate." More practised words! "I think her family would have been very ashamed, both for her and themselves, and perhaps preferred to deny they had any responsibility for her, though that's very sad for her little boy (or grown lad as he'll be now). He'll have nowhere to pay his respects. I cannot show you her grave, but, again, I know whereabouts she is. And she's not far from your mother. We can go together on Sunday afternoon if you care to."

She makes it sound like a picnic outing.

"And we'll take Aggie. She will like the fresh air and the trees. She arrived the same day as Ruth, I believe. And maybe one day Liza will be well enough for you to take her."

My heart is broken. Something inside me has shattered. "Why was I never told of these burials at the time? Why was I never allowed to say goodbye?"

"Death was common; it was not felt important. Poverty…" She pulls a face.

"So if you can find my mother, can you find my baby?"

"I have tried."

"Why? Without telling me…" I can't breathe.

"I have tried, but I cannot trace him."

"Why, what right did you have to search for him? And without saying owt to me? I looked up to you and Liza but neither of you ever really cared. I was 'just another lunatic' but wi' a baby. Just another case for you to study."

She shrugs. "We were all victims of circumstance."

"Ah, big words for excuses." I stand up as tall as I can, and go to the door. "But you will take me on Sunday. And you will *not* take Aggie. You will not hurt *her* as well." And I march out of the room and back to my bed, where I cry and cry, the tears soaking my pillow, the doll clutched in my hand, until Aggie comes to stroke my hair and the night bell rings.

VI

THE FOLLOWING MORNING I AM AWAKE EARLY. I feel lightheaded and empty from all the crying. As if I've been fed through the wringer like a bed sheet, and hung out tossing in the wind to dry. I sleep-walk to the kitchens and wait to be given my tasks for the day. Chef is cheerful. "My wife is going to have a baby!" he announces. I find it hard to raise a smile, but he doesn't seem to notice.

"How is the recipe book coming on, Mary?"

"I don't know. Can I show you sometime?"

"Of course, 'specially if it'll cheer you up."

I start chopping apples. They are last year's, stored in the larder, and their skins are dry and wrinkled and the flesh soft and pulpy, but they smell good, like the last days of summer, and they will make the pork and potato and onions in the stew for dinner go further. And some of the sloes I collected last year from the hedgerow by the goose field, and bottled with this in mind, will cut through the fatty pork and the apple sweetness as well. I am beginning to feel better.

I can see the sun shining in through the high windows of the kitchen, so I am surprised by the rumble of thunder. But then a siren sounds. I think it must be from the colliery across the valley. When you walk up to the hospital chapel you're at the highest point, apart from St Peter's Church, in the whole area, and you can see the winding gear in the distance, across a valley where they've built an electrical power station now, with great tall cooling towers. They never were there when my brother and I went foraging, but the coal mines were. We kept well away from them, we didn't like the men who came out of them, all black from the coal dust.

The siren's too far away to be from the village, and it's not the hospital alarm. It must be the mine. You get used to the whine of the siren at the beginning and the end of the shifts there, carrying across the valley, but this is different.

It keeps howling, like a dog howling at the moon. I feel as if icy fingers are crawling over my skin and it's giving me goose bumps. There must have been an accident. Sounds like the hospital fire engine is going out. I don't suppose we'll have our own engine much longer: it's not "economical", and it's hardly ever used.

Was the rumble a shaft collapsing, not thunder? I hope there's no-one caught down there. That would be worse than being cut off in the tunnels under the hospital. I were always frightened a bomb would trap us down there in the war. I am shivering. It'll be black as pitch down there, and surely icy cold. Should I pray for 'em? Or count my blessings? My hand rests on the warm scrubbed wood of the table I'm working on, and I remember what I'm doing.

Will the sloes be too bitter? Happen they'll not. This is one of my own recipes. You can do loads of other things with sloes, and they don't cost nothing. Like elderberries.

I turn to reach for a knife and something in my pocket

knocks against the table top. It's my old wooden doll. I found it on the floor this morning beneath my bed. I still keep it hidden between my sheets. I don't know why I brought it with me this morning. Perhaps I'll rub a little beeswax into the wood, to feed it and soften it. It's the only thing I can say that's truly mine.

Ah, thank goodness, the siren has stopped wailing. I look round. The kitchen is bustling. The door is open and people have gone outside to see if they can see or hear anything. Some of the girls are sobbing, one lass is screaming: her man were down the mine today. Chef has sat her down and is giving her a cup of water. He sends a couple of the other girls off to find out what's happened.

We all look a bit shaken up, I think it's the sound of the siren, it gets into your head. Like the sound of the bell in the tower here they used to ring when anyone escaped. I hated it. Thank goodness they don't do that anymore. The water tower, the bell, the chimneys; all standin' over us, watchin' us, guardin' us, but that bell, 'twere like a death knell. But this is worse, for, to be sure, it may *be* a death knell, a screaming, whining toll o' the Devil. And it seemed to go on and on for ever.

When I'm finished here today I must go and make my peace with Liza. 'Tis not her fault she's ill. I must remember whatever terrible madness made her kill her own child, it was caused by her illness. She needs me.

So, was *I* ill when I came here? Did having a baby make *me* ill?

I shall never understand this. Is Mabel ill because she talks to her sister? Is Doris ill because she's suspicious of everyone? Was Ruth ill because she was sad? Some of our ladies talk to themselves, or hear voices, or believe they are Mary Magdalene, but they don't seem ill to me. But if outside these walls people feel we need to be locked away, is that for their good or for ours? What would they think of me? We used to be frightened, when we were children, of the people in the asylum, but that was because we didna' know them and we were kept quiet with stories of the "loonies" escaping and runnin' off with us. Is it easier to say we're ill than to try to understand us?

I know there are some as can be dangerous on the back wards, will attack you if you look wrongly at 'em, and there are some as have fits that need watching all the time, but I think some are in here just because nobody wants them. And we look out for each other here.

"Don't we, Mabel? We look out for each other. Can I have those potatoes you've peeled? They need to go in the pots with the meat and the sloes. The apples'll go in last thing."

The kitchen is quiet and calm again.

After the meal's been cooked and served in the dining room, or sent on trolleys to the back wards where the patients can't come to the dining room, we do the washing up (as ever, the nurses won't let anyone leave until the cutlery's been counted) and then we can have our dinner. I am pleased. The sloes did work, and they gave some colour to the rather pale stew, but the apples just melted into the mix, too old and soft. The girls from outside stop to prepare our tea (usually not much more than bread and jam these days), but I can leave.

Before I go, though, the girls who went off to find out what happened down the mine return. They are flushed and excited, and they talk very fast and all together so it's difficult to make out what they're saying.

"It was one of them old shafts collapsed."

"No miners down there, it was a party of engineers, sent down to survey the tunnel."

"See if it could be opened up again."

"See if it were safe."

"Collapsed on 'em."

"Took so long to reach 'em, seemed like forever."

"We waited with everyone at the top."

"Brought blankets and thermoses of tea for when they got them out."

"And stretchers for them as were hurt."

"Cheered when they brought first one to the surface."

"There were just one left they couldn't reach."

"He were dead when they got there."

"Soaked to the skin. They cut his jacket off of him to try and warm him up but he were long gone."

"His mam came."

"She took him up and cried."

"It were pitiful."

"Then she said…"

"Yes, just real calm, it were a bit weird.

"But she said it loud, so as we could all hear."

"Surely, I were blessed… thou were never mine."

"And she took the towels and the blankets off of him that they'd used to dry and to try and warm him."

"And she cradled him in her arms, and then…"

"Naked thou came from thy mother's womb, and naked shall I return thee. The Lord gave and the Lord hath taken away. Blessed be the name of the Lord."

"Then the vicar went over to her and he said, 'Amen.'

"And we left 'em to their sadness, as everyone else wanted to sing and dance and cheer for the lads as had been saved."

"So we crept away and most, I think, went to the pub or the village hall."

As they finish their talking they quieten down and we are all still and silent. The tears are running down my face and I am crushing the doll so hard in my hand it is cutting into me.

Another mother, another son. No-one should die alone like that, not Ruth, not my mother, not that young man.

As I go I say to Chef I'll bring my recipes tomorrow for him to look at. He puts his arm around me and that feels comforting. I think there are tears in his eyes as well. "Take care, Mary."

I must go back to the ward to collect Aggie, and take her up to Ward 14 to get Liza but that young man will live with me for a long while yet.

And mebbe that's why I did go out with Molly to visit those graves, though, that one Sunday afternoon: Ruth's and my mother's, and all the others as had died in the asylum.

I met Molly at the entrance to the administration block and we walked around the bowling green to a door in the hospital wall. Molly had a key. On the other side was a road with little terraced houses such as I remembered from when I were a child. The road was cobbled and it didn't feel at all strange, but then we walked down a ginnel to a bigger road with newer houses and it all began to feel very different, and my heart started pounding. It weren't far up the hill the other side to the churchyard, though, and once we were there I felt calm again.

"Come, Mary. These are the newer graves; you can see the dates on the gravestones. We must go down there, to the corner. The graves are round here somewhere."

"I can't see owt but weeds and leaves."

"Look, take this stick. We can clear away the leaves with the sticks, and, see here, there's the outline of a plot. And there, that looks like a stone." I knelt down and used my hands to scrape away the weeds and moss that covered it.

"There's writing on it but I can't read it, it's been worn away."

Towering above us were enormous high trees, and the hedge had gone wild with blackthorn and holly.

"It's very dark and quiet here. Am scared, Molly. 'Tis a very lonely place to be buried. Are you sure 'tis right?"

"Yes, there are records with a map. It's difficult to say exactly where they are but definitely both Ruth and your mother are buried somewhere in this area. I will go and sit over there. There's an old bench. I think it will take my weight."

She left me to go and sit on the bench.

I was kneeling on the ground and my knees had sunk into the cold wet soil. I cleared a few more of the leaves away. Memories of my mother, of my brothers, of my childhood blew through me like an autumn wind; I felt the needles in my chest and the weight of my baby in my arms again, and from somewhere deep inside me I ached to reach out to my mother and have her hold me again. I needed her to know my baby, to hold him and sing to him like she did to Sam, and I stretched out and lay on the ground, my face against the earth, my arms reaching out, the closest I could get to her, my hands digging into the soil, and just for a minute, through the pain and the emptiness, I thought I could see her, sitting under a high window with the sun shining on her hair and my baby in her arms. And I thought she looked up and smiled at me, and I dug my hands harder into the soil and squeezed the stones and the wet earth through my fingers. And I just wanted to stay there for ever, for the emptiness and the anger to go away, for the tears to come and be wiped away, to go back to the day they took my baby from me.

I don't know how long I lay there, but it started raining and I realised how cold I was. I got to my feet again and brushed the dirt and leaves and moss off my coat and face as best I could with muddy fingers, and went to find Molly. She were waiting for me, lost in thought. I almost thought she were asleep.

"I'm ready to go home," I said, and started off toward the path, leaving her behind. Without a word she rose and followed me back to the hospital. I was still angry with her. How could she care so little that we might mourn our friends and family? Just because we were "lunatics" did we have no feelings, no rights? But she said nowt, and when we reached the hospital again she stopped at her door, turned and looked at me, sighed and touched my arm, then left me, again without a word. And I had no words for her, no words at all.

VII

AT THE END OF THAT TERRIBLE DAY IN THE kitchens when there was the accident in the mine, Aggie and I went up to Ward 14 to collect Liza. She had the smell of the paraldehyde on her. They must have had to give it to her to calm her down the previous day. She were untidy and sleepy, and her hair were all tangled and unbrushed. I think they must have put her in one of the padds for the night.

Sister was even more tightly buttoned than usual, and I could see why: the table that usually pinned her ladies in their seats had been removed, and the nurses were fighting a losing battle to confine the "wet and dirties". The ward door was still locked, and there was still little for the ladies to do, but there was a little bit of me that were smiling inside and wanting to cheer the ladies on in a bid for even greater freedom. But then we're all used to doing as we're told and we rarely question it, so I made no comment.

"Come on, Liza, let's go walking." And we set off. Yesterday had been a bad day. Liza had lost ground, but I felt sure we could regain it. I would get her out of that ward if it was the last thing I did.

I put my arm through hers, and Aggie trailed behind us. Liza didn't speak.

"Say something to me, Liza. I'm sorry you were upset yesterday. I'm sorry I was angry with you. I thought you were beginning to get better. Please speak to me again."

"I have nothing to say."

"Tell me about Broadmoor."

"Aaaahh, well, the grounds were very beautiful."

"Were there trees?"

"Trees and grass and flowers. We could surely walk out if we were good, as a reward, you know."

"That's good, Liza. Tell me more."

There was a long pause and she said nothing more for a while. We kept walking.

Soon we reached the cricket ground. The pavilion was all locked up but there was a bench we could sit upon. Liza and I squashed up to make room for Aggie, and I found a piece of string in my pocket to make a cat's cradle. This was a game we all knew. We took turns to make the string into new patterns until we reached the point when no further new pattern was possible.

"The string is like our lives," I laughed. "Whatever we do with it we always end up in a knot when we can go no further."

"But when we pull it off our fingers," Liza replied, "it always unravels and we're back to the beginning again. That's not like our lives at all! The moving finger writes…"

"And having writ," Aggie finishes it off for us.

"Moves on. Nor all thy Piety nor Wit,

"Shall lure it back to cancel half a line…

"Nor all they tears wash out a word of it."

"But we cannot be looking backwards all the time, Liza. You used to work in the sewing room, you did good work there. Perhaps you could sew again. You could make beautiful things."

"I did that in Broadmoor, hemmed 'kerchiefs for the Superintendent, and 'broidered them with letters. I still have nimble fingers, but sure 'n they shake too much these days."

We all held our hands out in front of us, and Liza was right, hers trembled and she couldna' still them.

"I had a great dream, once, but I cannot go back. I am too old now."

We were quiet again for a while.

"What happened to your baby, Liza?" I had to ask her, I could not let this hang in the air between us any longer.

"No-one knew, Mary. To be sure, I didn't know myself. I wouldna' believe it. It shouldna' have happened. I couldna' be expectin'. Then one night I got the pains, and they lasted all night, and all the next day, and then he came... in the bed. And I knew what to do for I'd seen me mam bring babbies into the world. But the voices in me head say he is a punishment. A good Catholic girl and married I should be fillin' the world with babes. For his little mouth were cleft and he couldna' suck, and when I laid him on his back he couldna' breathe. So I told the voices I would not have him, and they would not have him neither, and I put a pillow over his face. For he woulda' died anyhow. I surely helped him on his way."

I put my arm around her. She was shivering.

"But I still see him, like I see Ruth. And sometimes they speak to me and I cannot get away from them. And sometimes it's your baby as I put the pillow over. And sometimes it's your mother as tells me I shall go to Hell and burn in the everlasting Fire. For sometimes I think your mother died because of me."

"Oh, Liza, she were ill from the munitions. You told me that. How could you have..."

"Wicked thoughts, wicked words."

"No, Liza, she woulda' liked thee, but she were too ill. But I'm glad you told me about your baby though. Did you never give him a name?" I remembered how it felt to hold my Peter, the love inside me. I was sad Liza never felt that. "Come, we'll fight your voices together. And Aggie will help with her singing. Remember what you told us about being strong. We shall be strong. We shall stand straight and tall and fight them all."

So we stood up from our bench and walked back to the ward, and we sang together as we walked, but I cried for my baby and for Liza's baby, but I didna' let them see me cry, for that were *my* sorrow, and I could not share it; for neither of them would have understood the dreadful emptiness in the corner of my heart that our talking had opened up again.

But time moves on. Liza begins to smile, Sister Matthews leaves, the door to Ward 14 is unlocked, and the ward itself smells a little better. Some of the ladies are still confined to the ward, and there are still no doors on the lavatories, but sometimes people even speak to me when I go for Liza.

One day we go to collect Liza and I cannot see her. A little nurse glides up to us. I have seen her a few times but never spoken to her: she is new. "You look for your friend? I will find." And she glides off again, as if she were on wheels. She is very tiny, with thick black hair tied into a plait that reaches down her back to her waist. She brings Liza back to us and smiles.

"This is Priya," says Liza. "She is from India. You could be learnin' some things from her, Mary. She makes sweets that she brings us, like I've surely never tasted before."

Priya smiles again and disappears. I am bewitched.

"I don't think she's a 'proper' nurse," says Liza. "I think she's a 'nursing assistant'. The proper nurses give her all the dirty jobs to do and, Jesus, Mary and Joseph, sometimes I don't think they're very kind to her. She don't speak very good English and sure I've heard 'em laugh at her. Some of t' other patients are unkind as well, and I've seen 'em shout at her and spit at her. But we all on Ward 14 like her as she brings us those sweets, and cigs as well. And she makes me smile."

She is the first nurse we've had from India, though we've had a few from Jamaica. I really want to talk to her, but after that first meeting she seems to keep away from me. Sometimes I see her walking the paths through the old vegetable gardens to the door in the hospital wall, but she turns her head away. But I cannot get her out of my mind. One day I see that there is a man waiting for her the other side of the wall. It must be her husband. He is very tall and, I think, very handsome. Perhaps he is a maharajah. I've read about them in the encyclopaedia.

Maybe leaving the hospital would be no worse than leaving your home to come and live in a foreign country. I have looked on the map. She must have travelled thousands of miles. Maybe I should think about it some more. But I couldn't leave Aggie, or Liza at the moment. They have said to me in the past that Aggie shouldn't really be here. She should be in a hospital for "sub-normals" as she doesn't speak and she doesn't understand anything, but they kept her here because they didn't really know what was the matter with her: she gets so agitated, and then she will scratch and kick and bite, and scream and scream, and she was settled here anyway. I won't go anywhere without her now. It would be cruel.

But I think Liza is getting better. There is a new glint in her eye. She is having the electric shock treatment now. Each time she has it she sleeps for the rest of the day, and the next day she's very wobbly on her feet, but I think it may be helping. Molly says the electric shock is supposed to work like having a fit, and they started using it as a treatment because they noticed that some of them "epileptics" seemed happier and less disturbed after they'd had a fit. I can't say as I'd ever seen it, but the ones as had the most fits were always on the back wards. I'm glad there are better treatments for them these days, so there aren't so many in the hospital now. They had a hard time, with everyone being frightened of 'em an' all. Even some of the other patients thought they were possessed by devils. And the smell of that paraldehyde they used to give 'em made your stomach turn.

I still go to Ward 14 every day to take Liza out, and we talk as we walk, sometimes with Aggie and sometimes not. "Come on, Liza, let's go through the orchard. That's nice to see you smile. What have your voices been telling you today?"

"They're not so bad today, Mary. Sometimes I am so confused by what they put in my mind I can't think straight, but today I am well. And sure, we'll be having a nice little chat, and you can give me back my *Mrs Beeton* as I'll be needing it when I leave here, when I've got that little guesthouse and I do them coddled eggs for breakfast."

"Oh, Liza, that was always what you wanted, wasn't it? Have your own little guesthouse."

"We worked so hard, Bill and me. We saved up and made plans. It were surely both our dream. Then he signed up and went off to France, and when he came back he wasn't my Bill any more. He drank our savings away, and then he'd come back from drinking and demand his rights. And I'd fight him off as we'd said we'd not have a baby till we were settled wi' our own business. Then he lost his job as they couldn't trust him no more, and I fell for a baby anyway, and all my dreams came tumbling down around me. Then the voices started plaguing me."

I listen as we walk. There are long pauses. I'm glad I haven't brought Aggie today. It would have been more difficult to take in what Liza is telling me if she'd been here.

Liza is talking about her work. By the end of the war she was managing the house for the family who employed her. The men had all gone off to fight and women servants had left as well, so all she had to do all the work were herself, a cook and a downstairs maid. And she had to be lady's maid as well as household manager, and turn her hand to cleaning when needed. She was working nigh on sixteen hours a day, with Sunday half day, and keeping rooms for her and her husband when he was demobbed as well.

"Before the war I was a member of the WSPU, Mary, the Women's Social and Political Union. We fought for women's rights, but all that had to stop during the war; no time! Then when the war ended I tried to pick it up again.

"But then I started hearing me mother telling me I never should have left Ireland and I never should have married Bill. Then there were other voices, but I didna' recognise 'em. And they were telling me I were wicked and I didn't know how to be good wife, or keep me money safe. And sometimes they'd all be talking together so I couldn't hear owt else. And they said I wouldn't know how to care for a baby.

"Now surely they're saying I shouldna' tell thee, but they're muttering, and I am strong today.

"Can you help me fight them, Mary? I won before, until Ruth died, then they came back, telling me I killed her, and they were going to kill me. Or that the doctors had killed her and I hadn't saved her. That I deserved to die. And it was all muddled up with Ruth's baby. It was like as she was going through what I went through with my baby but there was no end to it for her. I couldn't bear that she died. And the voices said it should ha' been me not her. But that wouldna' ha' helped her. It were the keenin' that the nurses didna' like though, that's for why they tore me off her and put me in the padd. Jesus, Mary, her soul may have gone to Purgatory, but it were only fitting her body should be properly farewelled, and there were no-one else to mourn her. But that's in the past, and now I will be well again, I will. Help me, Mary."

"I'll help if I can, Liza."

"Sometimes it all makes me so weary. When they won't let me alone. But they've been there since I were seventeen, and mostly I've coped wi''em. I'm still a lady's maid, you know, I'm still going to have that guesthouse.

"I didn't tell anyone about the baby, though, but Bill found me, and the baby were dead and cold under the pillow, and I took a knife and wouldna' let him near me."

"Come on, Liza, you have said enough." I can't bear to hear any more. "Matron has talked about moving you onto our ward. That will be good. Then when times are bad we can fight the voices together. But now we're getting cold. Let's take this path, down to the chickens. We must walk faster to warm up."

She is thin now and easily gets cold. Her hands are old lady's hands: all bones and knuckles and freckled skin. I am not so old, but we both could have been grandmothers by now, and Ruth as well, and Molly even, if the war hadn't taken her husband. I remember reading about the "Lost Boys" in *Peter Pan*: they might have been *our* lost boys, lost but never forgotten, and always regretted. Dropped from their prams and never reclaimed, leaving a hole in our hearts, and an empty space we can never fill.

"Liza, you and I are survivors. I never had a dream like yours before: life was just ordered, day by day, the same routine, but now I think I really am going to be an author. I am going to have a book published: me, a writer, can you believe? My recipes in a book like *Mrs Beeton*. Now just look at the cockerel, Liza. He looks like one of the doctors, strutting round telling the nurses what to do, and the hens are taking as much notice of him as the nurses do the doctors!"

"Let's go back, I think it's going to rain. We'll go and find Aggie. Take my arm again.

VIII

I THINK IF I AM TO LIVE OUTSIDE THE HOSPITAL
walls there are two things I need; an identity, and friends.
I think I shall have an identity as a writer, but my only
friends are Aggie and Liza. And Aggie is lovely, but it is
difficult to share anything with her, and Liza is getting better
but is still sick. I would really, really like to get to know Priya.
I feel she could be my friend. I just don't know why she avoids
me all the time. She has bewitched me, I am sure, cast a spell
on me, though I don't know why. Mebbe 'cause she is quite
beautiful, or p'rhaps it's the way she walks, or more like glides
along, but I think most I like the idea of the story she must
have to tell.

I have looked up India on the map in the atlas in the day
room, and I wonder where in India she came from, and how
did she get here? What does she eat? And was England very
frightening for her when she got here?

P'rhaps she knows the secret to living somewhere new. I
try to think what it is that frightens me so much about living
outside the hospital walls, and I cannot figure it out. Is it

the buildings? Is it having no walls? Is it *things* that I won't understand, like machines? Or is it people; will they think I'm strange, laugh at me, or be angry with me?

I've never thought on friendship before. Never needed friends when I were a child, there were just me and Tommy and then me and me ma. Didn't need owt else. And in here? I found Aggie and that were enough. Though I s'pose Liza was my friend, and Ruth, and Cook, if having a friend is to care about 'em and know they care 'bout you, and you can tell 'em anything, and you know they're not perfect but you can care for 'em anyway. I just think if I had friends it would feel safer "outside".

And the "identity" bit? Well, it would be like a shield. People couldna' laugh at me if they could see I were "someone" or "something", not just a "lunatic", could they?

I am lying in bed trying to understand. 'Tis not easy when the bed's so lumpy. They changed our horsehair mattresses for sprung ones, but they're no more comfy. And they squeak when you turn over, and when you bounce on 'em, which is funny sometimes, but sometimes a bit shamin'.

But today is a special day. Today Liza is moving to our ward, and today I am going to talk to Molly and Chef about my book.

I have shown my recipes to Chef. He laughed at some of the ways I said things, but in a nice way. He is very happy just now as his wife has had a baby boy. Sometimes he sings in the kitchen, which makes *us* laugh at *him*. I think it was because he was in such a good mood that he tried a lot of the recipes out himself. There were a few things he changed, but mostly he liked them.

Then I tried typing them on the typewriter in Molly's office. I've done some of them but I was ever so slow, so Molly finished them off. And there's one of the patients does some nice drawing. That occupational therapist has been getting him to help with some art classes. He's a 'voluntary' patient in one of the new admissions wards, so they'll be hoping they can treat him and send him home quick, but he's done some nice little pictures for me of borage flowers, and tea cups, rose geraniums on a window sill, and rowan berries, and little pastries, and a roly-poly pudding. Chef thought they'd make nice "illustrations".

But I have no more time for thinkin'. Must be getting up.

I go on thinking about my book though all day, till the afternoon when I go to Molly's office.

"This project is coming on nicely." Chef is in good spirits, and even Molly is smiling.

"I think we need a little more text, a bit of introduction and a few more recipes perhaps. And we need a title. And perhaps some advice on growing some of the ingredients.

"I have shown what we've done so far to my brother and he's happy, with a bit of editing, to publish it. And he knows someone who's a "household name" whom he thinks will write, as a favour to him, a "foreword" to it."

"What about some more recipes then, Mary?"

I have an idea. "There's an Indian nurse on Ward 14. She makes sweets for the patients and brings them in. They all like them but they're different from anything they've had before. Perhaps I could talk to her and see if her recipes could be adapted for English housewives to make. That would be interesting and fun."

Molly frowns. "That young woman is a liability. And she is NOT a nurse. She is simply an assistant: unqualified and unregistered."

"What does that mean?"

"Every day she is a source of complaint or criticism from someone. She fraternises too much with the patients, she brings presents in for them, she undermines the nurses' authority. The staff complain about her, and then her husband comes in and complains that she is being harassed because of her race. And your Liza is whispering things to her about unions and rights and bullying. She is a troublemaker steer clear of her, Mary."

"She don't look like a troublemaker to me."

"Nevertheless, you may not speak to her. And Liza, thank goodness, is moving from Ward 14 to your ward. Why does that woman always get under my skin?"

"Who, Liza?"

"Yes, Liza. Every time I try to see things from her point of view she undermines me. These foreign nurses…"

"We need 'em, Matron," Chef interrupts. "And before them, many of the girls came from Ireland. Can't get more 'foreign' than that! At least Jamaica and India are not battlegrounds for the anti-British. And the girls are hard workers."

"They are lazy and insubordinate. Why do you think they're such fertile ground for Liza to sow her seeds of dissension?"

"No, Matron, they are oppressed and abused. Listen, one day, to what your nurses are really saying: they speak from ignorance and prejudice. Because they're black they say they're dirty, because they speak in patois they mock their English. I had thought better of you."

"Be careful, Chef. Just because I count you among my few friends in here you do not have the right to judge me."

"Then listen to Liza. She knows when the institution is being unfair."

"How do you know? I've known Liza for many more years than you. She is a left-wing activist and an astute politician, when she's sane. She will do anything to overturn the established order.

"And, Mary, that doesn't change my mind. I will not have you colluding with Liza to champion the underdog in here.

This hospital relies on discipline, and I will not see it fall apart. Go. We will discuss your book again another day."

I leave as quickly as I can. Is Molly frightened of Liza? At other times I think she seems to admire her. But then she's the same with me. One day I am her pet, and the next "a silly woman"; one day she wants to see me "outside", making a success of my book and my life, and the next I just annoy and irritate her. But she has made me even more sure I want to get to know Priya.

IX

LIZA HAS BEEN MOVED TO OUR WARD NOW, and she is so much better. I think she is having less Largactyl, and she is less sleepy but she's still quite slow. It takes her an age to get dressed in the morning. But I can see some of the old fire in her. So I ask her what I should do about Priya.

"To be sure, she's a sweet young thing, and she could probably be doing wi' a friend in here. But what are ye wantin' of her?"

"A friend, an ally perhaps. I'm restless, Liza. I think I do now want to leave the hospital, but I'm frightened. These walls and the routines hem me in, but they make me feel safe as well. 'Tis people as worry me most, though, being stared at or laughed at for being strange. I think Priya would understand that; she has to put up with patients and nurses making fun of her. When I weren't in here no more it would help to know someone else 'outside' as well. But they won't let me speak to her."

"Well, you must stand up to 'em. I'll be for helpin' you if you wish." Her face twists as she speaks. That happens a lot these days, I don't think she can help it. Sometimes it makes her difficult to understand.

"'Tis more difficult to get to see Molly these days. They stop you from just walking up to her door."

"We will wait."

We have to wait on benches in the entrance to the administration block, as I predicted. It hasn't changed much, but this part of the hospital still looks shiny, with the woodwork and the floors polished and the tiles and the paintwork gleaming. Our wards just look shabby now, and the airing courts, where Liza still likes to walk round and round, are wind-blown and uncared for, with the flower beds all gone to weed.

Finally we see people coming out of Molly's office and shortly after we are allowed in. Molly is sitting behind the desk.

"What is it you want? Be quick, I have a lot of work to do this morning, and, Mary, you should be in the kitchen."

"Matron, Mary wishes to meet with the Indian nursing assistant on Ward 14."

"I know and I have said that's inappropriate."

"Why, Molly? You want me to leave the hospital, but you won't let me meet someone who might help me with living outside, with my book."

"She would *not* be a good influence on you."

"Goodness, I am not a child anymore."

"Jesus, Mary and Joseph, what makes her a bad influence?"

"Liza, you know as well as I do. Her values, her standards, are not British values. She comes from a nation where there is religious divide and little Christianity, where there is dirt and disease, and poverty and overcrowding."

"That don't mean she's any the less for that, that she don't have a culture and a history of her own. You are prejudiced,

171

Matron, just as you were set against the poor white girls back in the days…"

"We have to maintain standards."

"So it's all right to employ them in menial roles, but they mustn't mix with the patients, infect them, pass on bad habits?"

"Mary is vulnerable. She needs to learn about the real world, not some fancy, imagined foreign one."

"I am learning, Molly, I am learning fast. I think the world out there must be worse than ever I thought." Molly has stood up. Her face is red.

"You are unkind and unfair." I feel the tears coming.

"Sure and you live in a strange world an' all," Liza chips in.

"I grew up when the Empire…"

"Sure ye did, but now the colonies are shakin' off their overlords. And their peoples are our equals, and you shouldna' be looking down your nose at 'em."

"I do not regard them as inferior, just different. And I will not change my mind about the Indian woman."

"Think again, Matron. Think again. 'Tis in your hands to lead. Would ye defend your 'lunatics' against prejudice? Would you have 'em part of the community? Then do the same for others as are 'different'. To be sure difference is a good thing, and black hands are not dirty, and niggers' hearts beat sweet as yours. But come, Mary, we have had our say. Surely we'll be gone now."

And Liza pulled me out the room before Molly could say owt more. In the corridor she stopped. "You wait, you'll be seeing your friend for sure now. Matron's no fool. She'll think on what we've said, just you see," and she smiled a sort of wicked, crooked smile at me.

And, of course, she was right, as Liza always was. It were not long after and it were Chef as told me: Priya and her husband were to visit me one day when Priya wasn't working in the hospital.

So one Sunday afternoon one of the nurses, I think her name was Bridie and she were Irish, like Liza, took me to the dining hall. We were not allowed to use the nurses' Christian names now but I'd heard them call her that and I thought it were such a pretty name. I was beginning to look at the nurses differently. I used to think that, if we were just lunatics, they were just our custodians, but now I was thinking some, at least, had lives outside the hospital, and some were as trapped in here as we were. Behind those caps and uniforms were lives and stories.

"This is exciting, isn't it, Mary? Visitors for you. Have you ever had a visitor before? You must be a good girl for them and maybe they'll come again."

I sigh. I really *am* too old to be called a "good girl". I'm sure Bridie doesn't mean it unkindly, and I am used to it, but it is demeaning and infantilising. And anyway my mind is on other things. This has all happened very suddenly and I am nervous. I haven't spoken more than two words to Priya before, and I want so much to be her friend. I don't know why, but it's just so important to me.

As we walk into the hall Priya and her husband are sitting at a table. As he sees me enter, her husband stands. I feel my face growing hot: how nice to being treated as a lady. I take the seat opposite them. I have to concentrate on what they're saying as my mind is taken up with the idea of being respected. That's never happened to me before, but… I must be gracious.

"Thank you for coming to see me."

Priya is smiling at me, so different from all those days when she turned away from me when she saw me. What has changed? She's telling me her husband's name is Ramesh. He really is as handsome close up as I thought he was from a distance: very tall, with dark wavy hair and a lovely smile. His skin is dark as well, a bit like gravy browning after you've added the flour.

"Matron tells me you are writing a cookery book. You want to know how to prepare the sweets Priya brings in for the patients."

"If she's happy with that, I would like to try and cook them, and maybe change the recipes a little to make them easy for English cooks to prepare, and then include them in my book."

"My wife would be honoured."

"First you must put in your book how to cook rice. So it is soft, and, how you say? Fluffy. Not boiled to mush like potatoes. The British do not know how to cook rice." Priya laughs. "You can teach them."

She has a high-pitched tinkly laugh, which makes me smile, and she's right about the rice: when we have it in here it's either solid and stuck together in stodgy lumps or it's a watery "gruel".

"I have written down in English what my wife has told me. These are recipes for the sweets. She does not weigh the ingredients so I have had to approximate the quantities. You may find they need adjusting.

"If there are ingredients that are difficult to come by in this country we have suggested alternatives, like oil instead of ghee."

"Though you can make ghee from butter, you know."

"These recipes should all be acceptable to the Western palate."

"Jalebi and burfi we make for Diwali."

"What is Diwali?"

"It is our Festival of Lights. We have many feasts and festivals in our culture. We have included the recipe for puris as well. They are like little fried puffy pancakes that we eat with kheer, which is like your rice pudding. We eat those at Diwali as well."

"Will you tell me some more about Diwali? Mebbe that is something I could write about in the book.

"And your clothes are very pretty today, Priya."

"It is sari."

It is a beautiful rich red colour with flecks of gold thread running through the silky fabric. I would dearly like to reach out and touch it but I daren't. "I can't see any buttons or fastenings. How do you put it on?"

"It is all one long piece. You fold and tuck and wrap. I show you one day. It is simple."

"I would like that. And could Chef's friend, who's done the pictures for my book, draw it?"

"I'm sure that could be arranged, if you really want." Ramesh hesitates. "Though I think you would be better to write for English tastes."

"Why are your clothes and food so different?" I am curious.

Ramesh smiles. "India is a very different country. Sometimes very hot and dusty, sometimes very, very wet. Different things grow there."

"Would I like it?"

"I don't know. It is our home but we have left it. Britain is our land of opportunity and we shall soon be English. Our children, when we have them, will speak English, not Hindi, drink tea and not chai, and go to school and grow up in your culture and this community. We shall be so English we shall not be noticed any more."

"But I will still wear sari."

"Perhaps…"

"But how can you leave your home like that?"

"There are many paths up the mountain and they all lead to the same place. The only person who won't get there is the one running round the bottom of the mountain telling everyone else they're taking the wrong path. You just have to have courage."

I'm not sure I understand that, but I do think they're brave, especially Priya.

"Why did you come to work here, Priya?" I want to know so many things. I want to touch her hand; I want to play with the bangles on her wrist.

"We did not have much money when Priya first arrived here. I have a good job, as engineer in the dye works, but we want to buy our own house. We need money for that. The hospital is close to where we live now, so it is easy for my wife to reach. She can walk here. They advertised for nurses' helps in the local newspaper, and my wife is strong even though she is small. She likes the work now: she likes the patients, though she was frightened to start with. Not of the patients, but of such a big hospital. She feared she would get lost and she might not understand what she had to do. She has never worked before. When she was in India she stayed at home with her sisters."

As he says all this Priya sits watching him and smiling. *Why doesn't she speak for herself? P'rhaps she doesn't know him very well.*

"But tell me, how do *you* like this place?" he asks.

"It is *my* home." What else can I say?

"Will you come and visit me again? When I've had a chance to try these recipes, so that we can talk about them. And then you can tell me more about Diwali."

"We would be delighted."

We all stand up and Bridie comes over to us. She has been sitting by the wall while we have talked. Ramesh shakes my hand and then he shakes Bridie's. Priya puts her hands together and bows slightly. "Namaste."

For the first time I notice she has a red dot in the middle of her forehead, and I realise how very young she is, much younger than me now, and yet, I suppose, so much older in experience.

Ah, well.

Bridie and I go back to the ward. I sit down with Aggie and read through the sheets of paper Ramesh gave me. I plan how I will try them out with Chef. I think, maybe he talked some more to Molly and persuaded her to let me meet Priya. Or perhaps it was just what Liza said to her.

Anyway, now I have done the other writing we agreed I would do to improve the book, and the gentleman on the admissions ward has finished the drawings. Molly has sent what she calls "the first draft" to her brother, who is going to show it to someone called Marguerite Patten to see what she thinks of it. And we've decided to call the book *Simple Kitchen Garden Cookery: Cheap, Easy and Unusual Recipes for the Busy Housewife*. Now all I need to do is see about Priya's recipes. Though we'll have to redo Molly's "draft", or mebbe we can just add a new chapter at the back.

X

MY BOOK HAS BEEN PRINTED. MOLLY SEEMS to have forgotten our visit to her office and the argument about Priya: she has never mentioned it at all. She tells me I have to have a bank account so that the publisher has somewhere to send the money from sales. And she says I must have some proper clothes to wear when people want to meet me. Once again she has taken me under her wing, though I fear that's a rather claustrophobic place to be. Today she says she will take me to the bank in the village herself and we can walk there, so that is easy. I am still very nervous of leaving the hospital.

I can't get used to the clothes people wear. Mine are very baggy and shapeless. I think I would like to have some new clothes but I wouldn't know what to choose, and I'm sure I'd be laughed at. Still, the bank manager doesn't seem to notice. He's shaking my hand, and I do a little bob to him, then I feel silly. Flippin''eck, I ain't no serving maid now, and I don't think anyone curtseys now anyways. The things a lass has to learn! He asks me to sit down and gives me some forms to fill in, telling me that I will get a cheque book sent to me in the post. (What in the world will I do with that?) He offers me a cup of tea, and it comes in little china cups with flowers around the rim, on a tray with a dainty teapot, and sugar if I want. And there are little iced biscuits that I'd like to take back for Aggie, but I daren't ask.

He's telling me that if I leave my money with the bank I shall earn some interest, so it will get to be more. They have told me how much money they will pay me for each book sold, but it doesn't mean much to me. I can't get my head round the pounds and shillings. I've not paid for anything for so long. Molly has managed all the talking with the printers, though she's tried to keep me involved and to explain what's happening.

I think it's very beautiful, my book. It has a lovely hard cover with a shiny paper dust cover, and inside the line drawings, of chickens, and borage flowers, and roly-poly pudding, are really pretty. And a famous lady who has written her own books about cooking has written an introduction on the first page, about the "originality" and "economy" of my recipes. Molly's brother knew her and asked her to do that. He thought it would make people interested.

I've finished my tea and the bank manager is shaking my hand again. We walk out of his office and past the smirking girls at the counters. I remember to stand up straight. I am an author! But I shall be glad when we've crossed that road and walked up the drive to the hospital again.

Molly says, "While we're here in the village why don't we have a look in the dress shop?" She has hardly said a word up till now.

My heart beats very fast. I won't know what to do. I feel sick. But Molly walks purposefully toward the window, with its mannequins and rolls of cloth.

Inside there are two ladies. They are perfectly dressed with high-heeled shoes and cotton gloves on their hands. They show me rows of dresses on hangers. The materials feel so soft, and the colours are so wonderful they make me feel giddy. I am so glad Molly is here. The shop assistant ladies, though, are really nice. I expected them to be quite haughty, but they are very kind and patient. If they weren't I think I would have to run out of the shop. They ask me what it is I'm looking for, and they smile when I say I have no idea. But then I think to myself, I *can* do this, and I remember reading the *Woman's Weekly*, and what did it say? "A woman can't go wrong with a little black dress", so that's what I ask for.

The ladies go into the back of the shop and bring back some black dresses over their arms. "Here, we have this one. It buttons down the front. It's quite formal and I think you would need high heels to make the most of the pencil skirt. What do you think?"

"Or this one. This one has a full skirt and it's belted. The three-quarter-length sleeves are quite fashionable at the moment."

I reach out to touch the material it's made of: it's so soft and shiny the folds run through my fingers like water.

"And there's a little jacket to go with it. Would Madam like to try it on?"

They take me to a little room like a cupboard but with a comfy chair, and a long mirror, and a curtain across the front. And there are coat hangers for my hospital clothes, though I don't hang them up. I fold them and put them on the chair: I am ashamed of how grey and shabby they look. And my underwear as well, stained with age and worn thin and patched. Where will I find new underwear? What would I ask for? I don't know what to do. I want to get back inside the hospital.

"Would Madam like some help? Would you like some black shoes to match the dress? It would help to show off the dress to best advantage."

"Yes, please," I whisper as I climb into the dress, and she passes a pair of black shiny slippers through the curtain. "I have guessed your size."

Bless her, I would have had no idea of my size if she had asked me, and my ignorance would have shown me up. I don't know what to do now.

"Come out and show us," Molly calls. So I take one more look in the mirror and get ready to draw back the curtain. I am shaking, but the dress is beautiful, and it feels so good wearing it. I've seen clothes like this in the *Woman's Weekly*. Princess Margaret wears dresses like this. But my hair… and my legs…

Molly looks me up and down as I step out. "You must have silk stockings to wear with it. And what size are the shoes? I think you could do with a half-size larger."

"Do you like the dress, or would you like to try something different, Madam?"

"No, no, it's beautiful. Umm, it's just what I wanted." How sophisticated that sounds!

"It suits Madam very well, simple but smart and elegant, suitable for day or evening wear. But can I suggest a handbag? This one would look nice with it."

I return to my cupboard to undress, and slip my hospital clothes on. This is something I must talk to Priya about: what clothes does one wear, when, and how does one buy underwear? She may not know, but I have met with her a few times now and I know if she doesn't have the answers we shall laugh about it, and find a way to get them.

The lady assistants wrap all my new clothes up and put them in a pretty grey bag with pink handles, while Molly pays the bill. I cannot get my head round the prices, though I can add them all up quick as lightning.

But when will I wear it all? And where will I keep it?

As we walk back to the hospital Molly says she will keep the clothes for me in her office and I can wear them if I have visitors or I want to go out of the grounds to meet people. And she tells me I am to have visitors very soon. Someone from the local newspaper wants to come and talk to me about my book. But before that I am to have a "social worker", who is going to talk to me about moving out of the hospital.

She tells me all this in a flurry of words, as if suddenly there is no time. She has been quite distant with me all day, quite preoccupied. She hasn't smiled at all, and hardly spoken. I am used to her moods but I wonder what I have done to upset her this time.

It seems particularly important to her that I meet my social worker before the man from the newspaper, though I'm not sure why. But I agree, and then I think maybe I should ask her what's troubling her, for she has been kind to me today.

"My brother, Mary, my dear sweet baby brother, is in hospital. He is dying. He has had a heart attack and now his heart is failing. He is literally dying of a broken heart and they say they can do nothing more for him."

"I am so sorry."

"I must go and see him. There is something I must tell him. Perhaps it's not too late."

We hang the clothes in the cupboard in her room, and then she is gone.

XI

THE ARRANGEMENTS ARE MADE FOR ME TO meet my social worker.

She turns out to be a young lady who sits in the day room with me with a folder on her knee, her hair tied back in a ponytail, a bright pink woolly cardy round her shoulders, and a long pink and white scarf trailing round her neck. She starts the conversation, without even introducing herself, with, "Well, we've found a lovely place for you to live, Mary."

Well, I'm not having that. "Why? And who are you anyway? What *is* a *social worker*? Are you a *lady almoner*? Me ma saw one of them one time she went to the hospital with her chest. *She* just wanted to know how much money me ma had, see if she could pay for her treatment."

"I'm sorry, Mary. No, I'm not even a proper social worker. I'm just a welfare worker. I work for the psychiatric social worker in the hospital; you must have met him."

"Yes, I think he comes to our ward meetings sometimes. Can't really tell the difference from the doctors, only he's more interested in us than the younger doctors."

"Well, he's really there to help the doctors. My work is to

help people like yourself move out of the hospital. You're to move into a 'group home.'"

"I can't go without Aggie and Liza."

"They will come too: a number of you have been selected to move. There are ten of you. Some you will know, but some are from other wards. Most of you are ladies but there are a few gentlemen as well."

"But how can you tell me to move? You don't know anything about me. And I don't want to go." I can't breathe and my heart is beating too fast.

"You have been chosen by the nurses here, but I must get to know you now, as I shall visit you in your new home and make sure you're all right. The ten of you are considered to have little need now of medical help."

"I never did have any need of… I just had a baby."

"I know, Mary."

"I should never have been in here. Are there others like me? Being moved around 'cause that's what suits you now?"

"There are some who aren't thought to be ill now."

"But did they have babies?"

"Not many, Mary. We don't send girls who've had babies to mental hospitals now, haven't for a very long time. And even when it did happen they mostly went to the sub-normality hospitals, not the asylums."

"That ain't no comfort."

"But it'll be lovely, Mary. You'll have your own room, and there's a kitchen you can cook in, and a little garden. And there'll be staff to look after you all."

"But I really don't want to move." I am in a panic.

"I will take you to visit. Did they say Aggie was your best friend? She can come with us."

"What will Aggie do without the airing courts and the orchard and the kitchen garden?"

184

"She'll like her new garden, and there's a sitting room in the house with a television."

"But what about my job in the kitchens here?" I feel sick. I was getting used to the idea of moving, but suddenly it's happening and I can't bear it. I am too frightened.

"You can cook some of the meals in your new home. And anyway, your job here won't last for much longer."

I am angry with Molly. She has done this. She's been pushing me to leave the hospital, and now she's gone behind my back. And this silly girl won't listen to a word I say.

"We have set a date for you to visit to your new home."

"Do I have no say in this?"

She doesn't reply, just gets up. "See you next week."

When the day comes this "social worker" collects us from the ward and takes us to her car, parked in front of the administration block. She's put her hair up in a French pleat and she's wearing a pink coat today!

Aggie and I have never been in a car, and I am really surprised at how calmly Aggie gets in. I hold her hand. Thank goodness it's not far, or I think we'd both be sick, we go so fast. We swing round corners and stop suddenly in front of a low, square two-storey building. It's very plain with brick walls and square windows, and it's surrounded by grass, with a hedge at the front and wood panel fences round the back and sides. Already I feel like I've been wrapped up in a blanket and I can't move or breathe.

The social worker opens the front door with a key. Such a small key, as you can hold in the palm of your hand, not like the ward door keys, and then she leads us inside. "Doesn't that feel nice? All light and airy, and they've put some nice pictures on the walls for you too!"

I see cream walls and pictures of kittens, and an orange-patterned carpet leading to a little shiny kitchen with a lino floor and a tiny electric stove.

"And upstairs you each have your own room. Look, your own cupboard space."

"Aggie has never slept on her own. She'll be frightened by herself. She must have a bed in my room."

The social worker looks a little agitated. "I'm sure that can be arranged. But just look at the bathroom: you can have a bath whenever you want, and there are some bath cubes for you there as well. You'll really love it here."

I am not convinced, but it seems I have no choice. Even if I lay on the floor and refused to move they'd just pick me up and carry me. And if I fought they'd give me the p'raldehyde, I expect.

But before they move me I must meet the man from the newspaper. I am to see him in Molly's office, and to wear my new black dress. I feel a bit strange. Molly isn't there; another nurse (I think she's a "senior" nurse, in charge of summat as they think is important, I expect!) has taken her place. I suppose she must still be with her brother. The clothes are beautiful but I'm not comfortable: they don't look right in the hospital.

The newspaper man arrives.

He is very young, or is it me that's getting older? I remember not to curtsey. He takes his hat off and, despite his youth, I notice he is going bald. He unbuttons his jacket and I see he has a woolly waistcoat underneath, and a bow tie. He doesn't look more 'n eighteen, but I suppose he must be.

"How do you do, Mary. My name's Frank, and I'm from *The Guide*. I want to write a short article about our new local author. Your book has proved very popular. Do you mind if I ask you some questions?"

He asks me about my recipes. "I'm no cook, but I think I could follow your instructions, they're very clear. Did you grow up during the Great War? Did your mother teach you to cook?"

I explain about my mother, and working as a kitchen maid. Then he asks me how long I've been in the hospital. "Since 1926." He hesitates, and we talk some more about working in the hospital kitchens, and using the produce from the hospital farm.

Then there is a long pause, and finally he asks me, "So, do you mind, why *are* you in the hospital?"

I explain about the baby. He looks shocked. "But why are you *still* here?"

"Because this has become my home."

"But, Mary, I know this is the first time we've met, but as far as I can see you're no more mad or sick than I am."

"I was put here for my own good."

"It sounds to me as if you've been exploited for years, unpaid labour, keeping the system going."

Then I realise why they made me visit the new "group home".

"Ahhhh. But I'm moving out very soon."

He has been writing everything down in his notebook. He is a very earnest young man. I wonder what he will do with it all. He wants to take my photograph before he leaves, and the nurse says he may, if I agree.

Before he goes, though, he wants to talk some more about how I came to be in the hospital. He asks what happened to my baby. What about the father?

I feel desolate. I can't answer his questions. "They told me he would be adopted. I wouldn't find him. But I loved him, you know. I still have the doll they gave me when they took him from me. I can show you if you like."

"Would you like to find him?"

"Of course, more 'n anything in the world."

"There are no records," the nurse interrupts.

"Then let's write this story. What more can you tell me? His name?"

I tell him everything I can.

"This is a gem of a story. Maybe someone will read it and come forward with some information that will help you to find your Peter," the young man says. "I shall enjoy writing this one, glad we've got some good photos. If you get the doll we can take a picture of that as well, might jog some memories."

My heart is beating very fast. Could that be possible?

As a final thought he adds to the nurse, "And can you get me an introduction to some of the other patients here who might be prepared to tell me their stories? I think we could run a series on this, 'specially if they have as juicy stories as this one to tell."

"You would need their consent to publish anything, and you would have to disguise their identities. And, of course, what you wrote would need to be approved by the hospital administration. But I'm sure the doctors would also be happy to talk to you about modern theories of mental illness and the new treatments if you want to put things in context."

When he's gone she sits back down in her chair. "Well, Mary. Matron will be pleased by the outcome of this interview. It'll be nice to see something about the hospital in the newspaper. Something positive, instead of the usual scare stories; something about patients being normal human beings and taking their place in the community. I don't know whether that young man can do it; we'll see. But don't raise your hopes of finding your baby. He's ancient history, and he'll only be a footnote to the article."

The young man from the newspaper visits again. I am not allowed to see him alone so the same nurse "chaperones" again.

He asks me some more questions, and I try to tell him how frightened I am of leaving the hospital, but the nurse takes over and lectures him about the errors of "institutionalisation", a new idea, she tells him, come from America, that means that patients locked up become dependent on the place they're locked up in and more ill rather than less. At least that's what I think she says. Institutionalisation: that's a new word to me. I shall try to find out more about it. Did she mean that was why I am frightened of leaving the hospital – that I am "institutionalised"?

The young man is polite, but he wants to talk to other patients, not to the people in charge. He wants to write a series of articles on different mental illnesses, using us as "case studies". He says this is quite revolutionary, but his newspaper readers ought to know about the people who live in their midst. His editor is very enthusiastic about my story, and hopes there will be more as good, and they are optimistic that the article about my baby will bring results.

"And then people would love to read about that as well," he says.

"People need to know about what happens behind the walls they've always lived with. Some of them will be curious, and some of them will be sympathetic, but those that don't want to know don't have to read my column. Mental illness has been a taboo subject for too long. And lost babies make for very good copy too, the icing on the gingerbread for me!"

I am excited. The nurse is wrong: Peter is going to be the most important part of the story in the newspaper. But I can't really believe anything will come of it. It all feels very unreal to me. And it makes my heart ache again. My beautiful baby, a young man now. I try to picture him. Would he look like his father, or my father? I try to remember what *they* looked like, for they were both young men, even boys, when I last saw them. But finding my baby, it's like living "outside" – I want it, at least I think I want it, but, at the same time, it's just too frightening. What if he were ashamed of me? What if he hated me for abandoning him?

XII

WE HAVE NOT BEEN TOLD WHEN WE WILL be moved into our new home but Priya has said she will visit me there. She and her husband have moved house and she is expecting a baby. I am hoping I will get to know her better then. In the meantime she has taken me to Woolworths and Marks and Spencer and I have solved the conundrum of ladies' underwear.

For the present I carry on working in the kitchens, until one day Molly comes in with a copy of the local newspaper. I have not seen her since she left to look after her brother, but there is no mistaking her mood. She is very, very angry. "Look, Mary, you're famous!"

She throws the paper at me. Covering two pages in the middle is an article about "Asylum or Unjust Imprisonment", with my words quoted and my picture.

The article talks about "your local mental hospital" and "patients who have been locked away for decades." And it promises a series of follow-up articles about mental illness today and its treatment.

But mostly it talks about Peter. And there is a picture of my doll, and a request that anyone who may have information that might lead to finding my baby contact the newspaper.

"So the little tart, who seduced a boy not old enough to know what he was doing, is now the martyr!" Molly spits at me. "What gratitude is this for the care you've received here? What a maudlin piece of rubbish this young man has written, no doubt to your order."

"I told nowt but the truth, Molly. I couldna' answer his questions better. Why are ye so angry wi' me?"

"Did I not say we had searched for your baby but there were no records?"

"But someone might know summat that were not in the records."

"You were always a selfish and wilful child, from the day you wrote to my mother."

I put my hands over my ears as she slams the kitchen door and disappears down the corridor. I am shaking all over but I am too shocked to cry. Chef puts his arm round me; he has shooed the other girls away. Somewhere in the back of my mind the final piece of a jigsaw fits into place.

"I must go after her."

"Do you want me to come with you?"

"No, I'll be all right."

I find her in her office, her head on her arms on her desk, sobbing.

"What have you done, Molly? What have you done?"

"James is dead, Mary, my brother is dead. And it's your fault! Your fault! He was the father of your child. Did you not guess?"

"No, Molly, not till just now. You kept it well hidden. But I should ha' done, shouldn't I. But you cannot blame me for his dyin'. Did *he* know, was *he* part of your treachery?"

"Only in his last few days. Then I told him, but he was too ill to be angry with me.

"He loved you, you know. He called you his first love and no-one could live up to the stupid idealised version of womanhood he created out of that. I think he was as deluded as some of the patients in here.

"So he never married, 'saved' himself, and never knew he was a father. And I thought I was protecting him." She throws back her head and turns to glare at me.

"What from? What did he need protection from?"

"From the shame of it, from the destruction of his inheritance, from a gold-digging little kitchen maid. I don't know. He was just my baby brother. I loved him. I would not, could not believe he had fathered a bastard child. It could *not* have been his fault."

"So I had to be a monster?"

"Were you not? A scheming, amoral, child-seducing little monster."

"Oh, Molly, I were but a child mesel'. You knew that, you called me a child oft enough. But when did you find out?"

"How can I say? I don't know. It was a gradual realisation, a process of putting two and two together, starting with your letter and ending with James's late night wine-fuelled confessions of his backstairs seduction and his adoration of a silly kitchen maid."

"But you cannot *blame* me, and not for his dyin.'"

"He could have married a good woman who would have cared for him, made him care for himself, made him want to live."

"No, Molly, 'tis all a fairy tale, and tha' knows it. He couldha' found me if he wanted to. If he wasna' what you wanted of him 'twere not my fault. It were just easier to hate me." She has put her head in her hands and is sobbing again.

"But sometimes you didn't hate me, did ye? Sometimes you were kind to me."

"As time passed I tried not to be angry and I started to have regrets. After all, your child would have been my nephew. I tried to make amends. I tried to find your baby. I thought if I found him I could bring you all together."

"Sort of happy ever after, eh?"

"Then I thought if I could get you out of the hospital and give you a new life...

"But then when James died all the anger came back. He should *not* have died so young. It was all your fault. If you hadn't seduced him he never would have died of a broken heart. My brother, *my* baby, would have been my baby for ever."

"Oh, Molly. I shouldna' forgive you for this, mebbe I won't, what you've done to me and to my life. But I don't suppose, if your brother and I had known what you had kept from us, it would have made much difference. Leastways, that is what I shall tell mesel'. I cannot live with more regrets. The pain of losing my baby is too great wi' out that. One day, though, I *will* find my Peter, and then at least he will know the truth.

"But *you* have to forgive me, forgive *your* construction of my transgressions, and I cannot help you with that. That is your salvation. You have to know that I cannot be blamed for your disappointments, or you will go to your grave a bitter and twisted and lonely soul.

"I shall go back to the kitchen now. I have nothing left to say. Do not follow me. I do not ever want to see you again."

So I go back to the kitchens, where Chef is waiting for me. I tell him that one day I will explain what has passed between Molly and me, but not now.

I take the newspaper and read through what has been written.

Will someone know where Peter is? I wish... be careful what you wish for, they say. As for the article, I have become not "just a lunatic", but the apocryphal child who was sent to the asylum for having a baby. I am not real, I do not exist, I am a fiction. My true identity, and my book, have hardly received a mention.

Part III

Kittens and Community Care

I

1960

ALOT HAS HAPPENED TO ME SINCE "THE *ASYLUM* years". *I have kept a journal on and off since I first learnt to write, at first on scraps of butcher's block paper and later in exercise books or diaries I was given. One day, maybe, this will all become my own story book.*

In 1961 Enoch Powell made his "Water Towers" speech. He talked of the need to "eliminate" the old outdated Victorian mental hospitals, with their water towers and chimneys casting long shadows over the countryside. And he predicted how resistant they would be to their own destruction.

And he was right. If we, the patients, were institutionalised, how much more so were also the staff?

It was only years later that I realised the significance of his speech, though I read bits of it in the newspaper at the time. But Aggie and Liza and I had already moved on, among the first "inmates" to be moved to small group homes in the community. For what I regard as the unhappiest time of my life.

There is sad and there is unhappy. I have felt great sadness in my life. But sadness is a deep, cutting pain that relates to real people or events, and is the flip side to great joy or love. Unhappiness is the slow ebbing away of the laughter in your life, leaving a constant greyness, a dull ache for something you can't even define.

So there were no great tragedies in our new "Group Home". But we were like birds caught in a cage. Gone were the great high windows through which the sun would send long shafts of light; gone were the green-tiled corridors and the high ceilings; gone were the acres of land we could wander. Instead we had bright, anonymous little rooms with gingham curtains at the windows, rooms of our own, but, in a funny sort of way, with less privacy than it seemed we had in a thirty (or more)-bedded ward.

And there was so little to do. Yes, there was a kitchen, and we were allowed to do some simple cooking, but it was so tiny, all Formica worktops and lino, and a table with tubular steel legs, and a very basic electric cooker that couldn't even be trusted to bake a sponge evenly.

And there was a sitting room with a radio and a television, in which most of the "residents" spent their day. And a garden you could walk around in five minutes. And on Sundays one of the staff would take a group to church if they wished, and later, from time to time, they'd take us out for a "pub lunch", a miserable affair where we'd sit around and eat "chicken in a basket" or scampi and chips, and drink half pints of shandy, while the other customers watched us with distaste.

I felt I didn't belong here, but I couldn't think where I did belong. Who was I? Day followed day without any purpose. I longed to go back to the hot, steamy kitchens of the hospital. I longed for my own space. And above all I longed to get away from those pictures of kittens on the walls!

In the end, despite my fears, I had wanted to leave the hospital so much. It was going to be a new beginning. But it hadn't been. And that article in the newspaper had somehow set the seal on what I thought was going to be my independence. All the *people who had contributed to my growing sense of identity had disappeared and I had become "just that story in a newspaper", not much better than being "just another lunatic". Frank, who had written the story, came to see me to show me the letters the article had generated, but none of them interested me and the few references in them to my baby were unhelpful.*

I remember, as if it were yesterday, how it was.

The first group of us to move have all been in the hospital for many years, and the staff who move with us are the old nurses, but we have our own clothes now, and the nurses don't wear uniform.

Aggie is quite confused to start with. I try to make the routines as close to those she is used to, but the garden is small compared with the airing courts. I sit and talk to her, for I think she does understand some things you say to her, and just talking gently is calming, but the slightest thing disturbs her: the doorbell, someone entering a room unexpectedly, being presented with food she doesn't recognise. Then she falls back into her old patterns of behaviour, and will scream, on and on and on, with her eyes closed and her hands over her ears, which is very distressing and very wearing for everyone. The good thing is that the nurses seem to have an unending supply of pencils and paper, so we often resort to drawing circles with her. This still seems to help.

Liza is less distressed, but she is sometimes confused now. I think it's just that her memory is not so good, so she forgets where she is.

"Sometimes, you know, Mary, to be sure, I think this is the little guesthouse me and Bill were to have, and you be all our guests."

We are sitting at breakfast with one of the nurses. "Would you like to be our housekeeper, Liza?" she asks. "Maggie comes

201

in every morning to clean but we have to tell her what to do. You could do that for us."

"Would you have us 'play house' then, like children?" I am irritated.

"No, Mary, it wouldn't be playing. Liza could check with the other residents what they want doing and how things should be arranged, and make sure things get done."

"And could we have fresh flowers in every room downstairs? Sure Bill 'n me we were going to have flowers everywhere. Bill were going to grow 'em."

"Perhaps Mary and Aggie could grow us some in the garden. We could dig up some of the lawn for flower beds."

"Do you remember the flowers we used to have on the ward, Liza?"

But she doesn't reply. She has dropped the cup she was holding in her hand and the tea has spilt all over the tablecloth.

"Jesus, the twitches have run to me arm now. I can't even be holdin' a cup steady. To be sure, I'm sorry, though. I'll be after takin' more care. We can't be washing linen all the time."

"Those twitches of yours are no better, are they, Liza? I saw you fall on the stairs yesterday when one caught your leg. And your ankles are swollen as well. We must get the doctor to see you."

"Whisht ye. I amn't no invalid yet."

"Do you remember how we all used to bathe together, and how we sang the hymns? We used to have to hold Ruth up sometimes or she would trip and fall."

"Sure, of course I do. I taught you all to sing 'Dear Lord and Father of Mankind', so I did, 'twas my favourite hymn. Aggie still sings it for me."

"We didn't know any other songs but hymns."

"We should have a piano in here. Ruth could play the piano, she told me once. Our class of women never could do such things, but Ruth were a lady. She were special, ye know. Silk and lace when she came, and they gave her our long wool skirts and aprons, and she never did make a murmur."

"We knew so little about her. She wouldn't talk about her home or her husband."

"I loved her, you know. I would have done anything to have made her better, but she'd seen too many taken from her, and dyin' in terrible ways.

"But she could have helped me run my guesthouse. She had 'breeding', would have known how to entertain proper ladies."

"Do you not think she would have been too busy with her family if she'd gone home?"

"Mebbe. She must ha' a boy somewhere. Does he no ask after her, d'ye s'pose?"

Does mine? I think.

"In the morning I wake when the sun rises and lie listening to Aggie's breathing in the bed next to mine, you know. The curtains let the light in but I can't draw them, for anyone could see in. How different is that from the glass of the high windows in the hospital, open to the sky day or night, welcoming the sun or the rain?"

We are quiet, remembering.

They have given me a little school desk in front of the window in my room. On it sits the doll they gave me when I first went into the hospital. Inside it, if I lift the lid, I keep my notebooks and pens and pencils. Molly gave me a Parker pen I can fill with royal blue Quink (I keep a bottle in my desk) but I prefer to write with my pencils, which I share with Aggie. We have a little alarm clock beside my bed to wake us in the morning, and when we get up I help Aggie to choose what she wants to wear from the clothes she keeps in her chest of drawers. She keeps them all perfectly folded and neatly arranged and she's beginning to accept that some things need washing from time to time but that they will return.

How life has changed.

"Do the voices still mither thee, Liza?"

"Not so much. The doctors thought I could be stoppin' me medicine: ye know, the old Largactyl. I be thinkin' tha's what ha' given me the twitches, but they ain't gone away for stoppin' it. But the voices ain't come back, so that's for the good. 'Tis great, this NHS, doctors and medicines for free. They've given me some tablets for me heart, that's what makes me ankles swell. But they can't do nowt for the spasms and the twitches."

One morning, not long after this conversation, Liza is not at breakfast. Rebecca is one of the new "care" staff who are gradually taking over from the nurses, and she bustles about. "Tea, ladies? We have boiled eggs today," but then we hear her on the telephone. "We've called the doctor. We can't wake her this morning." And then the door to the dining room is firmly shut as unseen people come and go, and no-one tells us what is happening, until much later.

"Liza is not well. Her heart isn't strong and it's giving up on her," Rebecca tells us, sitting with us at the dining room table. I think I should cry, but the tears don't come. I cried too much for her when she were on Ward 14. She were never the same again. I reach for another biscuit to dunk in my tea. Aggie is writing her name and drawing on a piece of paper torn from a notebook. The other residents gradually get up and walk away.

"Where is she? What will happen to her?"

"She is in her room; you may go and see her. They wondered about taking her to hospital; they think she had a heart attack in the night. But she said no. She said if she were to die she wanted to die here. They have given her painkillers and things for her heart but she is very weak. The district nurse is going to call again."

I go to Liza's room and sit by her bed. I hold her hand. She opens her eyes and smiles at me. "Sure, I never believed I could be so tired, Mary."

"Then you should sleep and get your strength back."

"No, Mary, I am surely dying." She keeps trying to catch her breath. "You are a good girl. Go back to Aggie and take the fight wi' ye. Remember what I told 'ee, ask those questions. Jesus, don't let 'em fob you off wi'out answers. Get outta here.

"Live, child, before it's too late. I didna' teach 'ee to read for nowt."

"Oh, Liza, I'm no child now." I smile.

"Surely you'll be always a child to me. But there is still time. 'Tis yourself as must find your salvation in this world. You bain't a lunatic now, but there's no-one else as will help ye."

She closes her eyes and struggles again for her breath.

"But forgive me, Mary."

"What for? I have nowt to forgive you for."

She is quiet. Then, "And forgive Molly."

"Why? What do you mean, Liza?" I speak gently and stroke her arm.

"We did not understand, not at all, at all."

"I were but a child then. You both helped me grow up."

"Indeed, indeed, but we could ha' been kinder. Ask her one day."

"Liza..."

"Go, now. I have no more strength, no more breath. I will sleep."

So I crept out of her room, and I never saw her again. The following morning when I got up her door was closed and all was quiet.

"She died in the night," Rebecca told me. "They said it was very peaceful. So sad; she was quite a character."

"She was my Liza, my friend. What will happen to her now?"

"Her body will be taken to the mortuary. Then they'll have to decide what happens to her."

"Will she have a proper funeral?"

"As far as I know she had no money or family, so I expect it'll be very simple. A pauper's funeral, no doubt."

"No, she must have a proper funeral."

"Well, if no-one claims her, there'll be no-one to pay for it."

"But I have some money from my cook book. I could pay for it. We must say goodbye to her properly. We loved her, and she cared for us, Aggie and me, and there were others as well. She were a Catholic, so it must be a Catholic service. But could she be buried in St Peter's churchyard?"

"I couldn't tell you but I'll get hold of the social worker; she might know."

"You know, Rebecca, I'm going to make this happen. I've done nothing, I've achieved nothing since leaving the hospital and coming here, but this is a puzzle I'm going to solve. What should I do first?"

"Don't ask me, I'm only 'care staff'. Never had anyone die on me before. Maybe you should just make sure you have the money?"

"How do I do that? Should I see the bank manager? I could walk into the village to the bank."

"You do that, and I'll talk to your social worker."

I went to the bank. Mostly you had to have someone with you when you left the house, but if you knew where you were going and they felt they could trust you they'd let you go on your own. At the bank they said I had to have an appointment, so I had to make one. But I told them it was urgent as I had to arrange a friend's funeral. Then when I saw the manager, he told me I had plenty of money for that sort of thing, and he wrote down how much on a piece of paper for me. And he told me I could use my cheque book for paying, and he explained how.

Then I saw the social worker, and she said she would look into what needed to happen and she would arrange for me to see the undertaker. It was all very difficult because I wasn't "next of kin", and it all took a long time.

When, at last, I met the undertaker, he was lovely. He was tall and gentle, and made me a cup of tea, and was very patient, going through all the things that needed to be done. The hospital had no details of any family, but he suggested we put notices in the local newspaper and the *Irish Times* in case her husband or her sisters were still alive and might see them.

He was worried about the cost of the funeral so I showed him the piece of paper the bank manager had given me, and he smiled and said that was very helpful. And we talked of coffins and handles and lots of other things which didn't seem very important to me, but then he said he would ask the Catholic priest to come and see me at the Home about the order of service, and the vicar of St Peter's to see me about the possibility of a burial in St Peter's churchyard.

The Catholic priest agreed to everything I asked, and believed it was possible for Liza to be buried in a Church of England cemetery, though he would need to officiate. However, the vicar from St Peter's wanted to know more. He sat with a cup of tea on his knee, and I felt as if my head were all in a whirl. I started talking very fast.

"You know there are patients from the old asylum buried in your churchyard, well, among them is a young woman called Ruth Atkinson, who took her own life. Liza loved her and never forgave herself for letting her die. That were long, long ago, but they must be together again."

"They will be, of course, in a better place," the vicar replied.

"Yes, but no, they must lie together, and Liza must have a headstone, and…" I could feel the tears running down my cheeks, and he handed me a handkerchief from his pocket. I couldn't stop crying, but he waited while I sobbed into his hanky and he drank his tea.

At last I took a deep breath. "And the headstone must read in memory of Ruth as well, as her grave is unmarked."

"We cannot dig your friend Ruth's remains up."

"No, no, 'tis sufficient they are lying in the same churchyard, if the headstone is properly written," I reassure him. He is quiet for a while.

"That is a sad little story. Someone else has been talking to me about a memorial for *all* the patients who are buried in our churchyard as well. Now the hospital is gradually emptying, people are asking questions about its past. I'm sure we can arrange for Liza to be buried as you request, and the undertaker will no doubt help you organise the stone. I have no objection to your adding Ruth's name; I do not think we need the diocese's permission."

I was so grateful I wanted to thank him over and over, but he said perhaps we should just sit quietly for a moment and say a little prayer for Ruth and Liza. Then he smiled and squeezed my hands and told me to keep the hanky, and he said I shouldn't worry: he would talk to the undertaker and the priest about tying the service and the burial together.

On the morning of the funeral I put on my little black dress and we found Aggie's favourite clothes, the long dark blue polka-dot skirt and white broderie anglaise blouse; and I brushed her beautiful curls and tied them back over her shoulders, and she let me kiss her cheek. Then I put the old wooden doll in my handbag, and took two golden chrysanthemums from the garden for Aggie and me to throw on Liza's coffin when they put her in the grave, for those were the flowers on the table on the ward that first day when I arrived in the asylum, though I didn't know the name of them then. Then we set off.

It were a grey day but the rain held off as we walked to the church following the hearse. There weren't many of us but a few of the nurses as remembered her came from the hospital, and Cook was there (I'd asked her, with her daughter. She were very old and frail now), and all the residents from our Home came, and a few of the care staff. The church was cold, but there were lots of flowers as I'd asked for, and an organist who played some gentle soft music. Then she played "Dear Lord and Father of Mankind", and I thought my heart would break as Aggie sang. And after, I stood beside the coffin and told Liza how we loved her and how she'd helped so many in the old asylum, especially me and Ruth and Aggie, and how we wished her peace now. And when I looked up there was Molly standing at the back of the church, but I didn't have time to wonder at it, though I thought she never liked Liza.

Then we took her to St Peter's and laid her to rest.

And went back to the Home and drank to her memory in warm Ribena in plastic cups. But I didn't speak to Molly, or see her again, and she didn't come back to the Home. The vicar did, though, and our social worker. She came over to me with a plate of little ham sandwiches Rebecca had made for us. "Mary, you did very well. It was a beautiful service and a lovely way to say goodbye to her. And you organised it yourself... you should be very proud."

"Liza always called me a child. I wonder what she would have said today."

"I think she would have said you'd grown up now."

"Maybe, or maybe she would ha' laughed and told me I'd got a way to go yet. She was never one to give up striving. But I think she would have been happy."

II

AFTER LIZA DIED I WAS DETERMINED TO find my identity again. But I felt lost. I tried to leave the building and explore the area we lived in. I started doing a little bit of shopping and experimenting with money, but I knew people were impatient when I couldn't work out what to give them. I spent time in my room practising with the coins and notes, so I recognised them, and my arithmetic got better. Then I bought a map and studied it. I found a coffee shop and bought myself a coffee and a cake. It felt very strange sitting in there drinking and eating, but, having done it a few times, I took Aggie, and she really surprised me by loving it, but that may have been 'specially because there was a ceiling fan in there that slowly rotated, round and round. I started writing again. I thought maybe if I could write a recipe book I could write a story, so I tried. That was my "identity", remember: I was a writer. And I started reading the books I'd already read again to see if I could understand how they were put together.

But it all felt very empty. I liked Rebecca and I could talk to her a little, but I felt so alone. I couldn't share anything with the other residents, not even thoughts about the things we watched on the television, though I did care for them all in a funny sort of way, as a part of my life, I suppose. But I couldn't call them friends. They weren't interested in any sort of discussion, and the best we could manage together was the occasional game of snap or snakes and ladders. I thought I had learnt to be self-sufficient, but I realised that I was really lonely.

Then one day the doorbell rang and Priya was on the doorstep. I could hear her asking to see me. I knew she had left the hospital to have babies, and I had heard that she had had two, one after the other, a boy and a girl, but I had not seen her for a very long time.

I was really surprised, but I ran to the door.

"May I come in?" She was wearing a sari with a woollen coat over the top, and pushing a big old pram with a baby inside and a little boy sitting on a seat on top. She looked thin and pinched, and cold, but the babies seemed really bonny. She stood at the door, hesitating, and I had to run out and drag her in by the hand. Initially she seemed quiet and a bit distant, but manhandling the cumbersome pram into the hall was such a bother we both had to laugh.

She took the little boy off his seat and he ran away into the sitting room immediately. Then she took the little girl out from under the pram cover, and the little thing smiled at me and put her arms out to be held. I took her so that Priya could take her coat off.

"Priya, you're so thin. I think you must have been neglecting yourself."

"I am all right. And look at the children, they eat so well. Ramesh is so proud of them. They are Paul, and this one is Ania."

They were indeed quite chubby babies.

"It is a long way to get here, I had to walk with the pram. I can't stay long, but I am too much on my own. I asked at the hospital where you were and they told me. I thought you might talk to me."

We followed Paul into the sitting room and I put Ania down to crawl. Paul had found an orange and was rolling it across the floor to Rebecca, who was on duty. Rebecca was smiling, and so were Faith and Elizabeth, two of the ladies who lived there with me, and who tended to spend their days half-asleep in the easy chairs in front of the television. Paul had certainly woken them up. We invented a game of "piggy in the middle", with Paul catching the rolling orange and everyone joining in, then Rebecca fetched beakers of Ribena. We were all a bit breathless from laughing at the game, but it had brought some colour into Priya's cheeks.

The children sat quietly while they drank their drinks and then Priya said she must go.

"You will come back and visit again, won't you? Next week? Which day? You promise."

Priya's visits soon became a regular thing. I was so delighted to have found my friend again that life seemed to begin to have some purpose once more, especially as now Priya needed *me*. To start with I would cook biscuits for her the day before she came: it was good to see her fill herself up with flapjacks rich in fruit and oats and syrup, and with sweet milky coffee. Then one day she came with a bag full of spices.

"Look what I have brought. Can I help you cook lunch? And we can make Indian sweets."

The staff were never very enthusiastic about my cooking. They had a set menu for the week, very bland and very boring, and they regarded my intrusion into the kitchen as "occupational therapy" at best and as a major accident risk at worst. Nevertheless, they were intrigued by what was in Priya's bag.

"Look, I have brought rice and vegetables." These she dug out from the bottom of the pram. "We can make a vegetable curry."

"We are having baked beans on toast with fried egg today. That's what's on the menu," said Rebecca, who was on "lunch duty" that day. "But I suppose we could do both and everyone can choose what they want."

There wasn't much room in the kitchen for me and Rebecca and Priya all cooking on the stove at the same time, but we managed. And Rebecca didn't bother with the eggs. Priya flew round the kitchen like a butterfly, frying this and boiling that and adding a pinch of this and a spoonful of that from the bag she'd brought with her.

By the time we sat down to eat Ania was asleep, but we put cushions on a chair so that Paul could sit at the table with us. Priya put the lovely fluffy rice on the table and a big dish of vegetables in thick red sauce.

"It is not too spicy," she told us. "I have not put much chilli. Please try." We all hesitated. Faith was bravest, taking some rice and a small piece of carrot from the dish to try. We watched, but we weren't sure what she thought of it from the look on her face. However, Paul was eating a bowlful of the suspect food with a spoon, and with great gusto, so we took our cue from him.

And we liked it. "It's really tasty!"

"Better than baked beans!"

Now even Faith was smiling. She'd wiped her plate clean with a crust of bread. "Can I have some more?" and Rebecca had removed the baked beans. Priya was laughing and clapping her hands.

"Can I come and cook for you again?"

"Oh, yes please."

So it quickly became a routine. Once a week Priya would come and help me with the little bit of garden I had dug up to grow vegetables and my beloved nasturtiums and borage. And then she and I would cook lunch for everyone. Gradually the staff were all won over by the different dishes we prepared, and the "residents", Faith and Elizabeth and Aggie and the rest, all looked forward to the day she came, though they had never tasted spices like these before. They were happy to entertain the babies, or be entertained by them, while Priya cooked. Even Aggie joined in: she seemed fascinated by the children, sitting watching them, even sitting on the floor rolling oranges with them.

Until...

A "manager" came to see us. He was a worried-looking little man with red hair and a quirky moustache, in a blue suit gone shiny at the elbows and a red tie as didn't really go with the suit.

"We have had a complaint from the neighbours. They have written a letter to the council and sent a copy to the local newspaper. See... here." And he put the correspondence page on the table.

"They say they are having to live with unpleasant cooking smells, smells of spices and onions and things. They say if they had wanted to live with 'foreign' cooking smells they would have chosen to live in Calcutta."

I am shocked. "It's only once a week, and why didn't they come and speak to us?"

"They never wanted 'mental' patients to move into their street in the first place," explains Rebecca. "They were already angry about that."

"We have already spoken to the staff and told them it must stop but I was delegated to speak to you, as this is your home. I'm afraid the cooking cannot continue."

"Why not?"

"It is already difficult enough getting planning permission to develop homes for people like you from the hospital in the community. We dare not jeopardise what we've got."

"That is ridiculous. But I suppose that explains why no-one ever talks to us or smiles at us in the street. We're still the 'lunatics' from the asylum. At least in the hospital we had our own 'community'. Well, if Priya can't come here to cook I shall go to her house. But it will be a sad day for everyone else here. Her cooking and her babies brighten everyone's lives."

"I'm sorry." I think he is sorry, but that doesn't help. I want to go and bang on their doors and tell the neighbours that they are cruel and unfair, but I know that wouldn't help either. Just confirm for them how dangerous we might be. "If they'd come to see us we could have shared some of Priya's sweets with them, and mebbe they wouldha' liked 'em, and they couldha' seen we're harmless."

So, as I threatened, Priya stops visiting and I start going to her house once a week to cook and talk and play with the babies. I am happy, but our "Home" sadly sinks back into its old lethargy.

Priya's home is a big old terraced house in a quiet leafy street. It is a lovely house with high ceilings and tall windows that let in the light like the windows in the old asylum. (Our Home is more modern and everything is small and square, with low ceilings, and part of the roof flat.) The first time I visit I go on my own and when I arrive Priya shows me into her front room.

"This is our best room… for visitors. Ramesh decorated."

The walls are covered in dark night-time blue wallpaper with a pattern of diamonds picked out in fine gold lines. There is a dark blue carpet on the floor, and the only furniture is a long dark blue velvety covered settee. In one corner is what looks like an altar or a shrine... not very big and about four feet high off the ground. It is decorated with figures in gold and red and other bright colours and seems to have little curtains draped around it.

"Can I bring you tea? English or Indian?"

"Where are the children?"

"They do not come in here."

"Then let's have Indian tea wherever they are."

Priya takes me into the kitchen, where she boils up tea, milk, sugar and spices, and pours it into small flowery cups. Then we go into the back room, where the children are playing.

"I am so happy you come here. Look, I make sweets for you. Do you like the chai? I so much miss my sisters. You will be my sister now. Come, sit on the floor."

We sit and Ania crawls over to us.

"I'll teach you to cook English food and you can teach me to cook Indian food."

"And next time you bring Aggie. It is a long walk, but you tell Aggie it's good for her. And I have a present for her."

"Aggie won't complain: she likes walking. And she likes you, and watching the children. She only complains if you try to change her routines without warning, or if something frightens her, and then she screams and screams."

When Aggie comes Priya gives her a big embroidered bag of bangles, all simple circles of brightly painted metal or glass. Aggie is enchanted, and lays them all out on the floor making them into elaborate patterns. We spend a lot of time sitting around on the floor. I find it strange to start with, and a bit uncomfortable, but soon I grow to like it. Priya laughs at me. "I shall teach you some yoga and you must practise every day, then you will be more flexible. See, Aggie has no problems on the floor, but I think she is what you call 'double-jointed.'"

217

"You must sit like Aggie, like this, and look with your mind at one point, like Aggie at the bangles. That is dharana. Then you sit with firmness and straight back and empty your mind of all bad thoughts, and you do not feel your body. That is dhyana. If you do every day you learn to be comfortable."

"Do you do it every day, Priya?"

"It is in my religion. To bring me oneness with the great soul of the world. It is difficult to explain."

"So it's like praying. We pray on our knees in church to God. I've never found that comfortable, however long I've done it for."

"No, it is not praying. We have many gods we pray to. But there is a great spirit that is in all of us and in everything. It is to become part of that.

"Look, this is Lord Shiva, one of our gods."

She shows me a brightly coloured picture she takes from another "shrine" in the corner. He has four arms and the moon in his hair.

"And this is Ganesh, the god of beginnings. I prayed for his help with my new beginning in England, and now he has sent me you, my new sister."

And she laughs and I can't help but laugh as well, but I rather like the god with the elephant's trunk. My God is a very stern god. I don't think this one would punish me for having a baby by locking me away for years and years.

"Our religion is full of wonderful stories. I will tell you some when you come. You will like them."

"What will she like?" Ramesh has come home and joined us.

"Stories of Krishna."

"And his sixteen-thousand wives! She'll not understand them. But I could teach you some maths and accounting, if you like. Tell you how public services are run, and what rights

218

and responsibilities you have as a citizen. I don't think anyone has ever told you those stories, Mary, have they? You might find them helpful. I had to learn these things when I came to Britain, though it was easy for me as India had copied many things from the British. I fear your hospital was even more a foreign country than India."

"I would like that, but I would like to hear Priya's stories as well."

"Then we shall start this evening. Come into the front room. I will put the gate-leg table from the hall in there, and Aggie can stay with the children. We will stop when tea is ready. I have a mind to start with mathematics and double-entry bookkeeping. That will help us to think about money and how to manage it."

"Have you taught Priya?"

"No, Priya has me to manage the money; she doesn't need to understand it."

"But..."

"No buts. Come. After that I will teach you about elections and what your local councillors do. We will make a woman of the world of you." And he puts his arm round my shoulder and steers me into the front room. Over my shoulder I see Priya disappear into the back room with Aggie, and I feel a little uncomfortable at having this special treatment.

So for a while each week when I come to visit I stay for tea, and, after eating, Ramesh and I go into the front room, and he teaches me for half an hour. Until the evenings draw in and it gets too dark for us to walk home, so Aggie and I have to leave before tea.

I learnt a lot, though, but in my heart of hearts I was glad when we couldn't stay. Ramesh was a good teacher and always very polite, but it seemed wrong to be sat with him while Priya was shut away in the other room. And I liked my time better with her, learning yoga, and talking about her family and her life in India, than the time with him.

However, one other thing that Ramesh did for me was to introduce me to the public library. We had had a librarian visit the Home regularly and bring us a selection of books, and we had been able to request books from her, but never before had I had access to such a wide range of reading materials. And I discovered poetry... or perhaps I just found it again, like a long lost friend, for when I buried myself in the verse the forms and the rhythms sang in my head as if they had always been there.

III

To introduce me to the library Ramesh takes me on a visit. We can walk from my Home.

The library is a very modern square building with a lot of glass. In front is a paved courtyard, which reminds me of the airing courts. Some lads are kicking a football.

"'Ere, kid," one of them shouts at me, though I'm hardly a "kid". "What ya doin' wi't' wog?"

"Get yr 'ands off her, ya dirty bastard."

"Fancy her, do ya? Go back where ya came from, and find you's own."

My heart is beating very fast and I can't breathe, but Ramesh just ignores them and keeps on walking. We go through the doors into the library.

"Don't mind them, Mary. They'll learn to trust us eventually. When they grow up with our children they will see we are no different to them. We have to be patient."

"But that was horrible."

"Sadly it seems to be happening more these days. When we first came in the fifties there were few of us and we were a bit 'exotic'. Now we are more, and we are beginning to be joined by our brothers from East Africa. And some are warning of 'immigrants' swamping British cities. But we are all from our great Commonwealth of Nations. We come with good will, skills to offer and new cultures to share. They are just frightened of us, and fear begets aggression, particularly in young men.

"But sticks and stones may break my bones, words will never hurt me: isn't that what you say?"

"Sometimes they were unkind to Priya in the hospital."

"But many are kind, as well. Assimilation, they call it. In time we shall all be one nation. This is the sixties, Mary, we have money, we have jobs, we have a future.

"Let me introduce you to Leah, she is the librarian."

"Ramesh, my friend." A tall, willowy young woman with long, wispy, sandy-coloured hair has come to the desk. "How nice to see you. Have you brought a visitor?" She talks with an accent which sounds American to me.

"This is Mary; she's not been to the library before but she likes to read. Can you show her round?"

"I sure can. What do you like to read?"

"I don't know. Jane Austen, Dickens."

"Ah, the classics. Have you read many modern novels? No? Well you'll find plenty here. They're in alphabetical order by author. You can take them home to read but you'll need a library card. If you fill in this form...

"And you could come to my classes if you want. The library has been given some money. We have 'an anonymous benefactor'. We've been told to use the money to run classes during the day on books and literature and reading and how to use the library. Would you like to come?

"There are lots of workers' educational classes as well, but they're usually in the evenings. But you could try them if you want. Now, though, there are lots of women at home during the day and they don't want to learn to be shop stewards; they want to learn for the enjoyment of it and to broaden their horizons. So they can help their children in school and be a bit more independent of their husbands.

"So we're going to give this a try. For two hours a week I'm going to invite people to come to the library to join a 'Literature Group'. I have a degree in English though I'm not a teacher, but we'll see how it goes."

"That sounds interesting," says Ramesh. "Perhaps Priya should go, but I don't know what she'd do with the children. Or perhaps I should go, but not during the working day." He laughs. "What about you, Mary?"

"But I've had no proper schooling. People would scorn me." The idea of going to any sort of class terrifies me.

"I don't think so. It's not a competition: people will be there because they enjoy reading. You enjoy reading."

So I went along to the first day. The class was much more formal than Leah made it feel when she first told me of it. The classroom was upstairs in the library, and we sat at rows of tables. It was full of young women, some studying for exams, I think, with a few young men sheepishly sitting at the ends of the rows. The first day I attended I sat at the back. We all had to say our names and by the time it came to my turn I was shaking like a jelly and could hardly speak, but the others were all much more confident. Leah wanted to know why we were here and what we wanted from the class. One of the young men made us laugh. He said he was an "actor", and he was "resting". He thought he might pick up some useful tips for auditions. I didn't like it though when it came to my turn and my voice went all funny as I tried to explain that I'd never been to school but I liked reading, and "Right dying swan we've got here," I heard him say.

Leah gave us a list of the books she thought we should read and told us how the sessions would be constructed. Then we started by reading a passage from *Tom Sawyer* and talking about the language the author was using. I didn't dare contribute but I really enjoyed listening. Leah seemed to like explaining things, and encouraging people to join in. I thought she must be ever so young: she couldn't be more 'n twenty-four or twenty-five, and she were wearing jeans. I'd never seen a woman in trousers before, leastways I don't think I had. But I thought she looked nice, and she had a lovely smile. She kept writing things on the board for us with chalks, and then she'd wipe her fingers down her jeans and leave white streaks.

Then halfway through we had a break and she came over to me. I had had to fill in a form about myself, though she already knew I had had no proper schooling, but I said I had written a book.

"So what's this book you've written?"

"It were a cookery book. It was published. I'll bring a copy to show you."

"Very good. And what would you like to learn by coming here?"

"I'd really like to know how to choose books to read, and how to get the most out of 'em when I do read them. And perhaps I'd like to do a bit more writing." I had no idea where that thought had come from! But it was true; I had tried a little already.

"Do you understand the proper use of grammar and punctuation?" She sat on top of the table, her legs crossed, leaning over to talk to me, her hair falling into her eyes. She were a bit plain, but she had beautiful blue eyes: funny, don't know why it should have come into me head, but they were just like my mother's. And she were wearing jeans again.

"Grammar? Not really. No-one ever taught me. What I've learnt I've got from the books I've read. It were easy wi' the recipes, I just followed the pattern in *Mrs Beeton*."

"Then when you go home why don't you try writing something for me, and next week I'll have a look at it. Come half an hour before everyone else."

"What should I write?"

"Anything. A Day in the Life of… My Favourite Walk… whatever, just not a recipe." Then she winked at me and stood up again, walking to the front of the room to start the class again.

At home I wrote about a day when Aggie and I had walked down to see the chickens with Liza when we were in the hospital, as I could remember the path as if it were yesterday, the may in the hedge and the cow parsley, like summer clouds, waving in the breeze, and I'd always loved watching the hens and the geese and making up stories about 'em.

Leah said she liked it, though she covered it with purple pen marks, correcting my spelling and adding in commas and semi-colons (I'd never used them in me life before!) Then she gave me more to do at home, suggesting exercises I could do writing description or conversation.

She started to ask me questions directly when I didn't say anything in class. I was so scared all those bright young people would laugh at me, but whether it was because she asked questions she knew I could answer or not, they never did. Unless I said something which I meant to be funny, and then they did laugh, and that felt as if I'd really become part of the group, and it were a nice feeling.

I still sat at the back of the class and I hadn't dared speak to anyone, but one day two of the ladies came over to me at the break. "We're Sally and Julia. Are you enjoying the class? We both find it difficult to keep up with the reading for these sessions. Don't you?"

I didn't really, but I didn't want to upset them. "Mmm. I do like the books though."

"We've both got husbands and kids, so there's such a lot to do when we get home."

"I can understand that. I have neither, so my time's my own."

"Do you live alone then?"

What should I say? How could I explain? Suddenly I felt very different from them all. "Not exactly."

But then I was saved by Leah asking the class to all move on to the next task, and Sally and Julia went back to their seats.

I wanted to be a real part of the group so much, but how could I be? Their lives were so "normal" and mine had been, and still was, so strange.

At the end of the class I asked Leah if she knew where I lived. She said she only knew I was a friend of Ramesh, who was a regular library user. She had my address but couldn't remember it.

"Leah, I'm what they call a 'long-term psychiatric patient' from the old hospital. That address sounds ordinary but it's a small group community home. All the people who live in it came out of the mental hospital. I shouldn't be coming to your classes."

"Why on earth not?"

"Because I don't fit in here." I could feel the tears starting in my eyes. "I don't have a family, I don't even look after myself really. I never went to school."

"Just look round the group: women chained to the kitchen sink and to small babies, an actor without a role, a shop girl who wants to go to university, a travelling salesman who is writing a play, and me, a failed Canadian poet turned librarian. Who's the misfit?"

"But how can I tell them?"

"Why do you need to?"

"They ask."

"I have an idea. How about if next week I ask everyone to write down something about themselves that could be the stepping off point for a short story or novel. I was going to do this exercise anyway at some stage to make people think about the process of writing. It will help our discussions to be a little more subjective for a while. Reading is the doorway to writing, but sometimes it's good to take a step over that threshold so you can look back from a different perspective. I will ask each person in turn to read out what they've written.

"You can tell them as much or as little as you like, so long as you're honest, and I'll support you if there are any negative comments."

So the next week I waited my turn and then, taking deep breaths to try to keep my voice steady, I read out: "I have lived most of my life in a mental hospital. I do not believe I was mad, but when I was sixteen I had a baby. My baby was taken from me, perhaps because I would not tell them who the father was. Then I was sent to the old asylum, where I lived, behind high walls, for some thirty years." You could have heard a pin drop!

I don't know what I expected. Pity? Sympathy? Horror? Disgust?

But mainly it was curiosity. "What was it like in there?" "What happened to your baby?" "What did you eat?" "Why didn't you leave?" All talking at once.

Except for the actor. "Little Miss Muffett likes to tell a tear-jerker, now doesn't she?"

Which made me blush as I realised that I had, indeed, taken centre stage, to use a metaphor better suited to our actor friend. In fact, I felt quite guilty that I'd hardly listened to what the others had said in response to Leah's request. I'd been so anxious about what I was going to say; I so wanted to *belong* to the group, but perhaps they did as well. I decided I would make an effort to understand their lives as well, and not spend my time being the "dying swan".

But I tried to answer their questions honestly. "It were comfortable, and it were safe. I learnt to read there, and I had a good job in the kitchens. They said I were there for my own good, and I suppose I believed them. I were what they called a moral defective. It were my home and after a while I never thought to leave."

"But you weren't a prostitute or anything, were you?"

"No, I were a kitchen maid."

Then Leah said she thought we should end the class there for that day, and as everyone left she came over to me and put her arm round my shoulders. "You did very well, Mary. You know you have a story there to tell. You should try writing it down."

As the sessions continued, then, I did try writing more; and I asked more questions, and answered more as well, risking being challenged, and confronting my fear of "getting it wrong" or being laughed at. If you never have to make decisions for yourself, I suppose, you never have to face these kind of demons. What does that make of you as a person?

Then at the end of the term we had a Christmas party. We went to the pub at lunchtime, and I wore my little black dress. It was still a lovely dress, though I thought it were probably now a little out of fashion, but no-one seemed to mind. It was very noisy and the "bright young things" from our class were all shouting at each other to be heard over "Jingle Bells", and "White Christmas", and they asked me what I wanted to drink, and I said "rum and blackcurrant", because I'd seen that on the television, but, my goodness it did make my head spin.

I asked Leah what Canada was like, and she had to shout back to me. "Very few people and lots of space… and just beautiful!"

"Will you go back?"

"Of course, when I'm ready."

"What will you do there?"

"Teach, I expect, and try to write poetry! I'm going to get myself another drink; do you want one?"

Then Julia and Sally came over. "What happened to your baby, Mary? You never told us."

"I don't know."

"Nothing at all? Did you not want to know?"

"Yes, 'specially when he was little. I missed him so much. But when I asked they wouldna' tell me. Then, as I got older I thought he would be grown and he wouldn't want me finding him. He mightn't even know about me."

"I couldn't bear not to know. If I lost my baby I think I'd die." Julia looked grief-stricken.

Sally put her arm round her. "Uh ha, even when they're screeching round the house pretending to be aeroplanes I love 'em, little buggers. Can't wait for 'em to go to school in the morning. But I'd miss 'em if they weren't there."

"Why don't you try and find him now?" Julia pressed my arm. "There must be records."

"But..."

"Even if he were adopted he might like to know about you."

"Though I suppose his new parents might not have told him about you, or even that he were adopted."

"But he hasn't come looking for me."

"That you know of."

"But don't you have the right to know?"

"Not by law, not if he's been adopted, she doesn't."

"Not ever?"

"Not ever."

"Just think, he might be tall, dark and handsome."

"And he might have his own children. You might be a grandmother."

"He'd want to know about you then, wouldn't he?"

"Go on, Mary, you must try and find him."

"'Tis not fair on him or you."

Leah came to join us. "What must she find?"

"My baby. They think I should try to find him."

"I'd be careful. Make sure it's really what you want to do before you start. You might find he didn't want to know you after all these years. Sometimes the past is best not explored. Sometimes it can be very painful."

"But would it be possible?"

"Well, did you say he was born in the old workhouse? Somewhere there should be records then. And his birth must have been registered. What was his name?"

"I called him Peter James Pearson. I told them that in the workhouse, but I didn't register him. They said they would do that." Saying his name made me remember, holding him, his tiny fingers around one of mine. I could feel the pins and needles in my chest again, and the emptiness when they took him from me. And I remembered the doll. I still had him, back "at home", sitting on my desk in my room.

I couldn't think any more. My head was spinning from the drink, and I wanted to go back to Aggie.

Then my friend the actor said he would walk me home as he was off to find himself some lunch anyway. I think 'twas the drink made me call him me friend. I didn't talk to him much in the classes. He weren't interested in writing. He just wanted to know the best way of "delivering" his speeches. Don't think he ever learnt anything, though, as he never listened.

I think he was surprised by where I lived. It looked like a council house, but too big for one: it had "institution" written all over it, everything impersonally neat and tidy, no toys on the lawn, no discarded gardening gloves or a favourite spade in the flower beds, no unmatching curtains blowing out the windows. I looked at it through his eyes, and cringed.

He stood at the gate and looked at the building, then he walked me up to the front door. I was still hanging onto his arm as I felt quite unsteady. But as he dropped my arm and turned to leave he suddenly put his arms round me and kissed me hard on the mouth.

I couldn't speak; I hadn't been kissed like that since I was sixteen, and not even then really. His tongue was in my mouth and I felt his knee between my legs, and his hand on my bum. I couldn't breathe and I tried to push him away, but he were too strong. And anyway I wasn't sure I wanted him to stop. I felt myself going limp in his arms and my body fitting itself against him. Everything was warm and wet and fuzzy, like it was with Aggie, but more so. My body wanted him, but my head wasn't at all sure what was happening. I just knew now that I definitely didn't want him to stop... but then we could hear someone coming to the door and he let me go.

"Sorry, Mary, I'm a little drunk, but you've been asking for that! Quite the little flirt!" And then he wished me Happy Christmas, and went off whistling to get some fish and chips. And Rebecca helped me through the door and I went to bed, though it were still the afternoon, but I couldna' lie down because the room kept spinning, and then I was as sick as a dog, and I swore I'd never drink rum and blackcurrant again.

Was that afternoon what they call a sort of "rite of passage"? I'd done "normal" things with "normal" people, even if I had got a bit drunk. Perhaps I were more "normal" mesel' than I thought. But I did wonder what it must be like to have a husband come home to you every night, and children to care for. Why had I never found my own baby? Could I have fought harder for him, and for me? Could I have had a family, like Julia and Sally? Could I have had a man in my bed o' nights? Was I a flirt? Was that how I'd come to be here in the first place?

All these thoughts, and more, went round and round in my befuddled mind; but worse, under all of them was the feeling that I couldna' escape, that I had made my bed and now I had to lie on it. That thought made me smile ruefully, given as how I felt at that minute about lying down, but it made me feel even sicker as well. I wanted to die, to curl up on the cold, hard tiled floor of the bathroom, to fall asleep and never wake up. I wanted all the things I had to face, the people, the decisions, the questions, just to go away. I felt as if I'd been dragged down into a great pit that had been waiting for me for a long time, a pit of shame and more; of guilt.

I finally got back to my bed and fell asleep with the taste of sick and blackcurrant in my mouth and the pillow wet with tears, clutching the old wooden doll to me again. I felt like I was hiding beneath the great bedstead in the ward again, and when I awoke Aggie was on the bed beside me with her arms around me. I wished then so hard we were back in the asylum again, where every day was the same, so you knew what was going to happen next, and people were predictable, and things didn't happen to you that you didn't know how to deal with, and you weren't asked questions you didn't know how to answer. But I wanted my baby again. I wanted him so badly.

IV

OUR DAY TO DAY EXISTENCE IN OUR "SMALL group home" changed very little as time went by, but a new staff member arrived, which was always interesting. Her name was Charity and she was from Jamaica. She was full of smiles and she would do things like putting her arm around Faith and asking, "Now where have we abandoned Hope today, then?", which Faith clearly found confusing.

Wherever she went or whatever she was doing she was always laughing and joking or singing. She sang hymns and gospel songs and Aggie followed her around soaking up these new songs. At first Charity didn't realise what Aggie was doing, but when she cottoned on she encouraged her and started teaching her part songs. Soon they were singing together, and Charity would be making beds or cooking tea with Aggie beside her, their beautiful voices, one deep and rich, the other sweet and high, filling our little rooms.

If she was working in the evening when the television was on and there was nothing else for her to do, she would come and sit with us and crochet. Aggie liked to sit and watch her.

Charity was very gentle and patient; she would slow down the speed of her hook so Aggie could see what was happening. She'd be making squares for a blanket in bright coloured wools, but, of course, each square started off as a circle.

Aggie liked to sit on the floor, as she'd learnt at Priya's. At first the staff told her to get up, but after a while they didn't bother. And it wasn't long before Charity had given her a hook and some wool and she was making squares as well.

We were at Priya's, though, when I learnt that Molly was living in a "Home" as well. We were sitting on the floor playing with the children.

"Do you remember Matron, Mary?"

"Of course."

"There is a man at Ramesh's work who is something to do with the old hospital, on a special board of something. I don't quite understand, but it was because of him I got work there. He told Ramesh that she had retired but she had gone to live in a special home for retired nurses."

I shrugged. "She was a strange lady. I think she cared about us but sometimes she seemed very cold and hard."

"She was very angry with the nurses if she thought they didn't care about what they were doing. We were all fearful of her. Many new ideas. The nurses were angry because they liked the old ways and thought how did she not value them. They did not – how is it? – see eye upon eye. It is easy to care for someone in a hospital, to keep them safe. But Matron said it was not kind."

"I don't know; was it not kind? It was certainly safe. I liked it better than where I am now."

"Then you must leave."

"Maybe."

"You know, Priya, the old hospital… I felt I belonged there. There was always someone would watch out for you.

No-one comes to our door now; no-one looks out for us. If Aggie screams in the street everyone turns their back. They don't speak to us, just write letters to the newspaper about us."

"I *belonged* in India. But I am here now. Sometimes you can belong to the wrong place. You have to make a new life, like me. And I have made two other new lives... and they need bathing before bed. How very *English* they are!" And she laughed, gathering Ania up in her arms and hugging her tight as she stood up and left me thinking on the floor.

It wasn't long before she was back, though, with Ania all warm and ready for bed and smelling of baby powder. She cradled her in her arms.

"No, Mary, I hate it here. There, so I've said it. I have been too angry to say it out loud before. I do not belong here. You and Aggie are my only friends. I must walk always where he tells me. I must be a good mother to his children, so they grow up English and learn and become rich. So they don't know how it feels to walk in the heat, in the dust, to bargain for the rice and the vegetables in the market, to step round the cows that get in the way, to dance with all their cousins at Diwali."

"But you are always laughing, Priya; you look so happy with the children, and so peaceful when you do the yoga. Don't you love Ramesh?"

"I am his wife. It is my duty."

"But what about the children?"

"Oh, I love them, but I am angry that they are not Indian, that he does not allow them to be Indian and Hindu."

"I didn't know you were unhappy, but perhaps I should have done, I'm sorry. I remember when you first came to see me at the Home. I should have known then. You were so pale and thin, and you said then you had no-one to talk to."

"Ramesh goes out when he's not working. I don't know where. Sometimes he comes back smelling of whisky. Then he laughs and jokes and teases me. He never talks to me even like he talks to you. He doesn't like me praying, and he not lets me mark our holy days."

Her cheeks are flushed but she has spoken softly and Ania has fallen asleep.

"Mary, I tell you because you are friend. You must not tell. Paul and Ania are my life here. And I try to love Ramesh. Maybe, one day, he will remember who he is and be proud again.

"But *you* must see Matron. She was part of your *belonging* in the hospital. She will help you belong outside."

"Mebbe, but what about you?"

"I am strong. I had four sisters. We had no brother. Our mother made us strong. She made us proud. And the yoga helps: it brings me close to them. But it is important to me that you are happy. Sad friends make sad company. I feel in my bones Matron will help you."

I felt, perhaps, she was right, and I should find out more about what had happened to Molly. A bit of me just wanted to forget her. Sometimes thinking about her brought back memories I would rather have forgotten, and vaguely disturbing feelings. It was a strange bond that had been forged between us, one that neither Molly nor I had acknowledged, for in a way we were sisters.

I had explained to Priya what Molly had told me about her brother, but Priya seemed to think that it was the time Molly and I had shared in the hospital that was more important to my identity.

So when I got home I did ask if the staff could find out more about her for me.

And that was why, one day, I was sitting on a bus with Charity, crossing town to a posh nursing home asking *her* about *belonging*. It had been easy for them to find out where Molly lived now, but they wouldn't let me go on my own.

"Where do *I* belong, Mary? This is my home now. I don't suppose I'll ever go back to Jamaica. But I don't know where I belong. I feel like I don't know who I am."

Charity was in her uniform with a thick blue coat over the top. My question made her look very serious, and she clutched her handbag tight to her chest.

"You know, when we first came to Britain, everywhere there were signs: no Irish, no blacks, no dogs. We used to joke, at least we're not Irish, and the British treat their dogs like princes!" She smiled once again, and gave the conductor the money for our fares. "Thank you." He smiled as well. He was also black. "It's getting better, though. In time we will belong.

"You know them gospel songs I sing with Aggie. They're not Caribbean, not Jamaican. They come from America. The hymns are ours, given to us by our English masters in slave times, but the gospel songs are from the slave times in America. But we feel we share that history."

I didn't know what to say. This was new history to me. I didn't really know anything about America.

"Our churches are growing here, and our choirs sing those songs, and that make me feel I have a sort of place here. And God loves us all."

But belonging must mean being accepted as well, and I was sad that people moved their seats away from us when we sat down on the bus. Why? Were they frightened? Did they think Charity's blackness would rub off on them? Maybe one day they'd enjoy the gospel songs as much as Aggie and I did.

I remembered how the patients used to spit at Priya and how the other nurses scorned her. I thought of how the people in our street turned their backs on us in our Home and wrote letters to the newspaper about us. "Would you let your daughter marry one of 'em?" That was the question they asked and so many said no. But mebbe Ramesh was right. If "our" children all grew up together they would learn to understand each other. Then they would fall in love and get married and all the prejudice would die. But that wouldn't help me and Aggie here and now, or Charity, or Priya. But I found it sort of comforting to know that it weren't just the "lunatics" that no-one wanted. The more people that were around as were "different", the more people would see as how "different" didn't mean "bad". *But glory be*, I thought, as I sat next to Charity on that bus, for that was what Charity would have said, *'tis takin' me a very long time to find where I belong, and 'tis definitely not in a "small group home in the community".*

The conductor broke into my thoughts and told us our stop was next, so we got up and stood on the platform at the back of the bus, holding on to the pole, the wind in our hair, ready to step off when the bus stopped. I didn't often do it, but I liked travelling by bus. When we hopped off I waved and smiled cheerily to the conductor, my little contribution to acceptance of difference, and then we walked along the pavement, under a canopy of leaves made by the branches of the big old trees growing beside the road, past big houses with fancy iron gates and large gardens, past neatly clipped hedges and perfectly cut grass, and past big cars parked in long driveways, until we found where we were going.

There was a sign with the name of the nursing home outside, and the entrance was up another long drive, lined with fir trees and laurel. We climbed up two wide steps and walked through thick, shiny, plate-glass window-doors into a room as big as all the rooms put together on the ground floor of our house, with flowers on a desk, a thick carpet, and long, elegant, sweeping curtains at the windows. It was very different from our Home, but then I knew Molly had plenty of money to pay for somewhere nice. And perhaps if you paid for it yourself you didn't have to have pictures of kittens on the walls!

After we'd explained why we had come we were taken to Molly's room, where she had a bed and easy chairs, a table and a glass cabinet with, I supposed, her own china in it. On the table was a half-completed jigsaw puzzle.

But I didn't have long to look round. She had called to me to come in when we knocked on her door, but when she turned to look at me (Charity had found a chair to sit on in the corridor outside) she did not smile.

"So it's you. What are *you* here for?"

I was taken aback. "I th-th-th-thought you might like a visitor. I thought you might like to talk again."

"Why should I ever want to talk to a patient again?"

"Oh Molly. I'm not just a patient, am I? You told me that. And you taught me to play hopscotch, and you helped me write my recipe book, remember?"

"You make a habit, I think, Mary, of invading people's privacy. And reminding them of things they'd rather not be reminded of."

"But we had some good times. It was where I belonged, the hospital. I thought it was important to you as well. I thought you might help me."

"Help you what? You're a grown woman now. You can take care of yourself."

"Then why did you come to Liza's funeral? I saw you there, but you didna' speak to any of us. But you hadna' forgotten us then. And when Liza were dying she said I must speak to you."

She turned away from me and was still and quiet for several minutes. I was standing just inside the doorway, just as I had come in, and my coat was beginning to feel too warm for the room. But then she turned back to me.

"Mary, I'm sorry. You gave me a shock. I didn't expect you. It was like seeing a ghost from my past." She was still not smiling.

"Come, sit down, I will ring for a cup of tea. And tell me what you've been doing. How is Aggie?"

I took my coat off and sat in the chair she pointed to. Then I told her about the Home, and my reading classes, and Aggie learning to crochet, but it wasn't what I wanted to talk about.

Molly softened a little and told me a bit about her life now too, so eventually I asked her again why she had come to Liza's funeral.

She didn't immediately answer again. "Perhaps I can explain one day, but not today. You may come back and see me again if you really wish. And I would like to see Aggie again."

"And once you said to me you had tried to find my baby. How?"

"Mary, leave it be. It was all a long time ago. It's past history. Forget it."

"But you said you couldna' find him. Why not? What did you do?"

"I simply looked for the workhouse records. But you will not find him. Let it rest, Mary. Searching will cause too much unhappiness. Go, now, I am weary. I will try to be kinder when you come next, but go now."

V

"LEAH, HOW CAN I FIND THE RECORDS THAT'LL help me find my baby?" I asked when I came back from seeing Molly. I found Leah at the library, in her office, searching through boxes of old books for something. She had her jeans on again and a big woolly jumper with a thick rollneck and sleeves pushed up to her elbows. This time she were wearing glasses which she pushed up onto the top of her head, into the hair she had plaited into thin little pigtails.

"I'm not sure, but Ramesh could probably help: he's a mine of information about that sort of thing. Let's talk it over with him," she suggested. "We could meet here at the library. But now, let's go and get a coffee, I'm fed up with these dusty old books, and I'm gasping for a drink." And she took my arm and led me out the door, waving to her assistant as she went.

There was a café not far from the library, which was good, as it was just starting to rain. We sat down at one of the Formica-topped tables and Leah ordered coffee and tea cakes.

"I really like a good cup of coffee, Mary, don't you?"

"I don't know, I hardly ever drink it. Give me a good brew any day. Do you drink coffee in Canada?"

"Yes, but tea as well."

I felt a bit awkward: I wasn't used to going to cafés. Leah took out a packet of cigarettes, lit one and passed them to me. "I'm so glad you came by. I am so fed up with this job. I am sooooo bored."

"Why do you do it then?" I pushed the packet back to her.

"Need the money. Can't move on till I've saved some. I enjoyed the teaching, mind you; that was fun. But I need to get back to writing again. But writing doesn't make much money, especially writing poetry." She tapped the ash from her cigarette off into the little tin ashtray on the table.

"What do you write about, Leah?"

"Mainly it's poetry. Can be about anything, but when I get back to Canada I'd like to write some fiction. Hoping I can use what I'm learning on my travels."

"Where are you going to go next?"

"Europe, I suppose, perhaps Scandinavia. I know quite a few people in Canada whose families come from Scandinavia. But I can't afford it yet."

The coffee arrived and she stirred sugar into hers. She looked so self-assured and sophisticated, but I wondered if she were a bit lonely. Where does she live? Does she have a boyfriend?

"I'm trying to write something about my life in the hospital, Leah. Would you help me with it?"

"Of course, if you want me to. I think that would be very interesting. We could meet at the library or I could come and see you at home. Bring something with you you've written about when we meet with Ramesh. And don't forget what I've told you before: show, don't tell. Use your imagination to make me feel I'm there too; don't just give me a history essay."

"I won't, and please do come and see me at home. I'd really like that."

I felt quite excited by our conversation, and I thought Leah was quite pleased as well, though she seemed to have forgotten it when we met again, this time with Ramesh.

"I don't even know my baby's birth date," I told them. "I know it was 1926 and I know it was September."

"We should be able to find his birth registration, and then we need to find the workhouse records. The old workhouse is now the general hospital, but they will either hold the records or know where they're stored." Ramesh was enthusiastic. He had said he would be delighted to try and help when I asked him. I was hopeful something would come out of our meeting, but I was uncomfortable that the three of us were meeting without Priya. I would have liked her to be there; she would have understood how I was feeling.

"How exciting! I've done a little reading about practices in the workhouses of that time. There's quite a lot of information archived here in the library. By 1926 babies like yours might well have been put up for adoption. From 1926 adoptions started to be registered, so that might make it easier or it might make it harder to find Peter, I'm not sure. I presume he would have been fostered immediately after he left you, possibly with a wet nurse? That should be recorded somewhere.

"Women who were paid to do that sort of fostering had to be registered. That came in in about 1908, I think. In the Children Act. I think it was a response to some cases of 'baby farming', where women had been paid to take babies and neglected or killed them. Sounds pretty horrific."

"Ugh, how horrible, but that were long before Peter were born."

"Yes, I know, but it does mean that if he was fostered it would have been with someone who was registered, and

243

therefore she should be identifiable. She could be still alive. She might be able to help us."

"What if he's been adopted? His name will have been changed."

"That, I admit, could be a problem."

"Well, let's see how far we get."

I wanted to go and tell Priya straight away, but I had to wait. I was excited but frightened as well.

Ramesh and Leah made plans about finding the records they spoke of. "You know, if we have no success we could try the *1939 Register*. That was like a census, but they recorded details of every man, woman and child in the country over one weekend so they could be given things like ration books. They used it when they set up the NHS as well."

"The problem with everything like that, though, is that the information is confidential, so unless you can prove you have a right to know you can't get access to it. I think it would only work if he'd died."

"Maybe this is going to be harder than we think!"

When I saw Priya I had to tell her about Molly as well as the search for the records.

"If it was meant to be, the records will tell you what you want to know. Ramesh and Leah are very clever. But you must go back and see Matron again. That is more important."

"Why?"

"I don't know, but it is. I feel deep inside me that she holds a key, or a piece of a puzzle. Like one of the bangles missing from a pattern Aggie has made."

Leah and Ramesh took me to people and offices in all sorts of places. Sometimes I felt they just took me because they had to, not because they wanted to. They worked so hard at finding the information they said I needed, but they didn't really talk to me about it. I felt it was a project they, and not I, shared. Leah said she found the searches fascinating, and then she started to talk with Ramesh about seeing if they could find information about her own family history too.

I liked Leah. She was always very helpful when I asked her questions about books and about writing, and now she'd promised to help me with my hospital history. She was a very independent sort of person, young and full of life and very "modern", with her jeans and her short skirts, her cigarettes and her coffee. But she'd never said much to me about Canada, or her family.

"Like a lot of Canadians, my family were from England originally. They didn't want to find their 'roots'. They didn't speak of 'the mother country' with any affection. I think they just wanted to forget it. And that's the way they brought me up, to be Canadian and to be proud of it. I hadn't thought of looking for my forebears before, but Ramesh thinks I should."

And I had always admired Ramesh. He, like Leah, was a good teacher, and he'd taught me a lot of useful things in our evening sessions. And he was very handsome. But I loved Priya, and I wished I could trust Ramesh, but there was something about the way he looked at Leah that made me feel uncomfortable. And why did Priya always have to stay at home?

In between all these visits and discussions, however, I found time to see Molly again.

I took Aggie with me.

Molly was more welcoming this time. She had a tin of coloured pencils and a book of drawing paper she gave to Aggie, who sat on the floor and drew some very beautiful and intricate patterns. Who would believe you could recreate the leaves on the trees outside the window, and the sun shining through them, out of circles of different shades and sizes, or perfectly represent a corner of Molly's room? The patterns

Aggie drew with her circles had gradually become more and more elaborate, and now were clearly pictures, and very accurate pictures, though they didn't contain a single straight line. And once she'd drawn something, she could repeat her picture, exactly the same, over and over again.

Molly made me a cup of tea, and showed me the copy of my recipe book that she had kept. "I've never been much of a cook myself; that's why I came to live here. All my meals are cooked for me. One of my sister's children came to see me the other day. I showed it to her, and she said *she* might try some of the recipes."

"I think they might be a bit old-fashioned now; foods in the shops are different."

"Some things never change. My sister died, you know. She was older than me. Her children still come to visit, though. I was sad when Liza died; that's why I came to the funeral.

"We never really saw eye to eye, but I came to admire her, too late to tell her so, I'm afraid. She was working class and my family were definitely socially in a different league. I felt she resented my money and my power. And I resented her attempts to undermine it. She was a very clever woman and, were it not for her mental illness, I think she would have made a name for herself.

"But I believed we had to maintain the social order. That's the way I was brought up, to believe that men were born to be leaders, not made. I couldn't be doing with her 'socialist' principles."

"I remember once you called her a troublemaker."

"I did indeed, many a time."

"Why did she go to Broadmoor?"

"I wasn't the only one that thought she was a troublemaker. And we couldn't stand her keening for that lass that died. She wanted to lay her out and she wanted her to have a proper funeral. It was easier to send her away."

"She should have had a proper funeral. Like me ma. It were cruel."

"I know, Mary, they were cruel times. I would like to make amends somehow, one day, if I can."

We were both silent for a while. The room were very pretty, so different from my room. And it were very quiet; you couldn't hear footsteps outside or anything. There were pink roses on the wallpaper and curtains at the window that matched. And I recognised the pictures on the walls, though the photographs were too small to make out.

"Didn't your brother paint the pictures?"

"Yes, indeed, my baby brother. I loved him as the child I never had. I just wanted to protect him. That's why I was so cruel to you.

"I'm sorry."

She were silent again and I thought we'd best leave. I picked up the pencils and paper and helped Aggie stand up from the floor. I said goodbye but she didna' reply. She just looked up briefly at us and there were tears in her eyes, but she said nowt.

But then I turned back to her. "What was it that Liza said I should ask you about? What other secret did you keep? What did she know that you didn't tell me?"

She got up stiffly from her chair and walked slowly to a small chest of drawers. Out of the top drawer she took a box.

"There was a day, after you had sent that letter to my mother, and I'd figured out that James could be the father of your child, when something happened. I was with Liza. We'd been asked to sort some linen, make an inventory and order some new supplies for the sewing room. We were doing it in the women's dining room. One of the clerks came to say there was a woman from the village who wanted to talk to someone in charge and they couldn't find anyone; would I do it. So I said they could send her in to me there. She was very nervous and she said she was in a great hurry and could not stop. She would not sit down. She said she had fostered a newborn baby from the workhouse, Peter James Pearson. She knew the mother had been admitted to the asylum, and to start with she had hoped the mother would be released and reclaim her baby. However, her own little boy had died, and she had grown to love her foster child. She thought she would try to adopt him. She had been told if she went down that road she would be forbidden to contact the baby's real mother. So she was very anxious. Before the little boy's name was changed for good she wanted to let the mother know that her baby was a strong, healthy and happy little boy who would be well loved and cared for. And she wanted her to have this photograph."

Molly took a picture out of the box and handed it to me. It was a very small faded black-and-white photo of a little boy in a dress such as they put babies in in the 1920s, sitting on a flat surface (could have been a table), looking very seriously at some wooden blocks in front of him.

I had to sit down. Was this my Peter?

"So why did I never have this picture? Why was I never told?"

"I told no-one. And I told Liza you were not to know. She was very angry and we had an argument. I was frightened of her, but I said if she told you I would tell everyone that she had killed her baby. A few of the nurses knew that but none of the patients. She didn't want that, and anyway I told her it would just unsettle you and there would be nothing you could do about it. So eventually she agreed."

"Did you know the woman's name?"

"I was told, I think, but I forgot. No note was made of it at the time. No note was kept of her visit. Liza never knew her name."

"But you said you tried to find him, my baby."

"Yes, I have many regrets, and one of them is that I never noted her name, for when I searched for the records of the foster placements from the workhouse the relevant ones had been destroyed in a fire. I have never been able to find her name anywhere. And I have tried everything."

"Did you show this picture to your brother?"

"As he was dying."

"Oh, Molly, what have you done? What have you done? How many people have you hurt? This was your nephew. My beautiful, beautiful boy, my son. What did he know of me?"

"I am sorry, but it is done and cannot be undone."

"You are a cruel and selfish woman, and I cannot forgive you for this. Come, Aggie, let's go home. I shall take the photo."

I took Aggie's hand, which, of course, she didn't like, but I had to get both of us out of that room as quickly as possible, get out into the fresh air and try to breathe again. Then we walked, for miles it seemed, till I got my senses back and found a bus to take us home. Then I put the photograph safely away in my little desk so that I could look at it again when I felt calmer. I would take it to show Priya. She was right about Molly holding a piece of the jigsaw that was my life, but I don't think it was the piece either of us expected.

VI

Back at the Home I started to write again.

I was sitting at my little desk one day in the room I shared with Aggie. They had put it there for me to write on when I first arrived, and then later I used to do the "homework" Leah set me on it. I still worked at it, though I was no longer going to classes. Leah had taught me verse forms and composition, and given me books to read, but words had a magic and rhythm of their own for me, and I'd used them to conjure up some poetry of my own. I'd even had a few things published. Now, though, I was starting to write the history of my time in the hospital, and I was hoping Leah would find the time to visit and help me as she had promised.

"Mary, would you like a cup of tea?"

My goodness they're employing children here now, was the first thought in my mind. "A cup of tea would be very nice, dear. No sugar, thank you." Why was the tea here always weak, milky and sweet?

A new lass had started working with us. She was seventeen and her name was Beth, and she came from a "Home" herself – a home for unmarried mothers and babies. They had found her this job as a care assistant.

She was a pretty little thing, with soft brown hair like mine, and long delicate fingers. She brought the tea in a mug that had a picture of a kitten on it... ugh! "Do you do a lot of writing?"

"Not a great deal, but I enjoy it. I once wrote a recipe book and that was published."

"I would *so* like to get something published. I have been writing as long as I can remember: stories, my diary, essays at school. What I'd really like to do is write a book for children, older children, about real live modern children, and what it feels like to grow up now. I've had a go at some short stories. Would you read them for me?"

"If you wish, but I can't say as I know much about growing up. I did mine in a lunatic asylum. How old is your baby?"

"She's four months and her name's Louise, but I call her Lulu."

I felt very cold suddenly and pulled my cardigan round my shoulders. "Are you feeding her yourself?" I remembered the pins and needles.

Her face flushed red. "Yes, it's hard work, but I can still feed her when I get back from here."

I drank my tea, while she sat awkwardly on Aggie's bed.

"And who's the father of your child?"

"Just a boy at school. He doesn't want anything to do with her."

"You must bring her in here to meet us."

"I can't do that. I have to leave her in the crèche at the mother and baby home when I go to work: it's the rules."

"Bring her one evening. You're allowed out, aren't you?"

"Yes, but…"

"We won't eat her. We've had babies here before. They're very popular!"

"Okay, I'll do that, if I can bring you some of my stories to read."

"A bargain."

A few days later she brought Louise into the Home. She seemed quite big to me, but then Peter was only newly born, so he would have been smaller as I would remember him. Her head were not wobbly, but she couldna' sit up yet. Beth handed her to me and I smelt the baby smell of her skin. I held her close to me. I couldn't let her go. She looked at me and wriggled and I thought she was going to cry. I thought I must smile at her but I didn't know how. Priya's babies were always older than this, somehow already independent little beings. This little one was still so fragile and tiny. I took a deep breath. "Hello, Lulu." Then I was laughing: she had my finger in her hand. She laughed back at me. We were friends and Peter was only a memory again.

"Now, have you brought those stories for me?"

I thought she had talent, but I didn't feel able to say more than that. I wondered if Leah would advise her. I was struck by the thought that I might be able to help her myself. But I needed to think about the implications. And I needed to get to know her better.

So I let time pass.

But with time came the realisation that our searches were not finding Peter. Leah and Ramesh had reached a dead end, and seemed to be losing interest. We found Peter's birth registration. Which was good, for it proved he was real. It was probably silly but sometimes it felt, despite his picture, as if he had just been a dream. But there had been a fire at the workhouse, as Molly had said, in which a lot of papers and documents had been burnt, and we could find no remaining reference to Peter or what might have happened to him. And all other possible avenues led us nowhere.

Every day that Beth came to us to work I thought of her and Lulu, and wished…

And every day I became more fond of her, but also more irritated by her.

"I was adopted as a baby, but I've fallen out with my parents since I got pregnant," she had told me. I was amused by the realisation that Beth is Elizabeth, born 1953! Did she get that name from her adoptive parents, or from her birth parents? Which set of parents were the royalists? I would ask her one day.

But in the meantime I felt she must meet Priya.

So I invited Priya to visit us at the Home again. She came and made chai and brought coconut ladoos with her.

Aggie liked the ladoos: they were sweet and sticky, and all perfect spheres, exactly the same size. Aggie had learnt so many new skills since people had made the effort to understand her. Priya had taught her some basic cooking skills, and Charity had taught her to crochet. And her drawings had become increasingly refined. I could see that she liked Beth; and Priya, who had a special bond with Aggie, also immediately wanted to hear all about Lulu.

As I watched them all together, the three people I felt closest to in all the world, I suddenly realised that I didn't need to spend the rest of my life in the care of social or mental health services. I *could* live independently if I wished. I could take on supermarket shopping, managing a bank account, caring for my own home. I just needed to make it happen. I should not be fearful. Fear was just the legacy of all those years being locked away: I could conquer it.

I did not need to belong in anyone else's world. I did not need anyone else's approval. Aggie was my love, Priya my friend, and Beth... well, there was just something about her, even if sometimes I could have thrown things at her, she annoyed me so much.

Part IV

High
Windows

I

1970

TODAY IS THE FIRST DAY IN MY NEW HOME. I am carrying a suitcase. It contains all my clothes and the few things I own, mainly notebooks and pencils, and, of course, the doll, worn and rusted but still with me. I walk through the little wooden gate (that needs a coat of paint) and up the path to the front door, my front door. I have two keys on the keyring in my hand and I use them to open the door. Inside is a long, dark hallway, a mosaic of red, brown, white and black tiles on the floor, brown tiles on the wall up to the dado rail, dark wallpaper above that, a single lightbulb hanging from the ceiling. I smile. This is really mine; I can make it my own. Here I shall welcome my friends. I put the suitcase down. (They lent me that from the Home. They wanted to bring me but I wanted to come on my own.) There are two doors off to the left. The first leads into a cosy little room with a fireplace and a bay window. The windows are tall and they let the light flood in from the street outside. In the middle of the floor, on the bare floorboards, is the desk, a child's school desk, they found for me to write on beside the window in the room I shared with Aggie. It was kind of them to send it here.

The second door opens into another bare room with a fireplace and high windows, but these are long narrow "French" windows that look out onto a narrow paved path leading to a small garden beyond.

The hallway leads then down two small steps to a tiny kitchen, just waiting to be warmed by a new cooker and filled with the smell of newly baked bread. I promise I will get you a new cooker, little kitchen, and we shall bake and roast and steam good things together. Though the cobwebs and the rust and the stains must go first.

Back down the hall and up the narrow stairs, and here we have a room for me and Aggie, with high windows looking out over the street to the park beyond. And, oh, in it are two beds, all made up with new sheets and eiderdowns, and Charity's crocheted blankets: I think Priya must have organised this. And there's an old wardrobe, so somewhere for our clothes, but no curtains or carpet. We can manage without the carpet but I think I will have to buy some cheap sheets to make into curtains as a temporary measure.

Back down the landing and here is the bathroom. The bath is a dreadful shade of shocking pink, but it will do, and then, here it is, my room. This is where they should have put the desk, by the window, where I can sit and read and write and think: perfect. I shall put the doll on the windowsill.

More stairs, to two rooms in the attic. These will be Beth's rooms, under the eaves, and already there is a bed and a cot in here. I bought them second-hand from a shop I found quite near to my old Home and Ramesh arranged for them to be brought here. And, dear Priya, she's put sheets on these as well.

I go back to the bedroom and sink down onto the floor next to one of the beds. There is a tree growing out of the pavement in front of the house, and its branches lean over to my window. Almost hidden by the autumn leaves there is a robin there singing to me. Liza's spirit, maybe?

How long has it taken me to get here? To get to where I belong? It has been a battle. Liza would have approved of my fight. I feel tired at the very thought of it, but there is much more to do.

When did I decide to start my own "belonging", to stand on my own two feet and declare my independence? My plans certainly didn't get off to a good start! You may well laugh, Mary Pearson: remember the social worker's face when she got wind of what you wanted to do? She had to interfere, and I didn't have the courage then to stop her! (My life has been so full of appeasement. How do I learn to say "no" now, at my age?) I remember the "sheltered" flats and housing schemes she took me off to visit. New ideas and probably good ones, but not what I wanted. Why shouldn't I sit on this floor? It's cold and hard and dusty, I know, but it's tiresome never being allowed to do anything that's not good for you. I don't want to live anywhere anymore where people will be forever telling me what to do and what not to do, telling me what's best for me.

So I will make my curtains from sheets, and I will buy myself the cooker I want, and I will cook all those recipes from your book, Liza (I still have *Mrs Beeton*). But I wish you were here to share it. And I wish I could have watched my little boy grow up somewhere like this.

I stand up slowly, pulling myself up on the bed. I shall paint all these walls light and bright, and Beth and her baby will fill the rooms with life and laughter, and we'll have a proper fire in the grate, and not a single picture of a kitten anywhere. And, if we have to have a shocking pink bath, I shall paint the whole bathroom pink and purple, so there!

Ramesh and Priya have been very helpful. When I said I wanted to find my own place to live Ramesh was full of advice. I didn't really want his advice but he was determined to help, so I made it a condition of our discussions that Priya be involved. Which was good, as we all sat on the floor in the back room of their house, with the children tumbling over us and Aggie making bangle patterns, and talked of renting rooms, of property prices, of mortgages, of good places to live... and bad. And we laughed a lot, and Priya added good advice, which I could see surprised Ramesh, and I learnt a great deal, but mainly that to get what I wanted would be hard.

Ramesh and Priya had bought their own house. "I had a good education in India. I was clever and good at learning. When I came here I worked hard and made myself valuable, so I got good jobs, so I could buy this house. But most people rent a place to live. Good places to rent are difficult to come by, though.

"Between the two wars, when you were safely tucked away in hospital, there were plans to clear the slum housing, the old back-to-backs and the tenements, and build new houses that anyone could afford. Then the war came and the demolitions and the building stopped."

"Ramesh, that's all old history," I would say to him. "It doesn't help me now, and anyway how do you know all this?"

"When you first come to a new country on your own you have to find accommodation. You learn. You are offered cheap rooms, sometimes for too much money. They take you to places where whole families share one room, where there are no proper bathrooms, toilets outside. You soon learn to avoid these places, but you do not forget."

"But you weren't in England during the war."

"No, but I came not long after. Even now, with new towns and prefabricated houses, there are not enough good places for people to live."

"I've read about the slums, and I've seen some of the old bomb sites in town. You'd think they would have cleared them by now."

"The future is bright. This 'land of opportunity' will conquer this problem. Harold Wilson will come back. He will build more houses. Soon there will be enough houses, enough good places for people to live, you will see, but for now it will be difficult for you. I tell you this because it was difficult for me, but now look what I have. You must have perseverance. I like that word. You do not need a nurse to tell you what to do."

"Ramesh thinks Mr. Wilson is Britain's Gandhiji!" Priya laughed.

"Mr Wilson is a good Englishman, a good Yorkshireman. I am also a good Englishman now. I listen to the news, I watch the television, I need to know about the land my children are growing up in. I need to know they will have good places to live, like you. You should have a good home of your own. With Aggie. Not a 'hospital-outside-of-a-hospital.'"

"Ah, Ramesh, I have a little money from my book, but not enough."

But then a strange thing happened. I received a letter from a solicitor in London telling me that I had been left some money in a will. It gave no details but the solicitor asked me to contact him. This I really didn't know how to deal with, so I had to seek Ramesh's help. And the outcome was that I found that I was suddenly quite rich, but I had no idea why, as the bequest was made on the condition that I shouldn't know who had made it. There seemed no way I could find out and I could think of no-one who would have wanted to give me such a great deal of money. Sometimes I would sit on the floor with Priya and we would try to guess, but our guesses were pure fantasy, ranging from the possibility that a hospital visitor had fallen in love with my food to my own personal dream that

261

Peter had grown up and made his fortune, and had wanted to make his mother "comfortable" without revealing his identity.

Wherever the money came from, it gave us a whole new set of concerns to mull over in Ramesh and Priya's back room. But it also made it possible for me to buy this little house. In one giant step I have become middle class, middle-aged (well, perhaps a bit more than *middle*-aged), and a home-owner. It feels very strange, and a bit daunting. But I'm here now. Liza said: ask a new question, face a new challenge, every day, and I'm certainly doing that. I don't even know how to buy paint, let alone how I'm going to get it on these walls.

I think this house must have been owned by someone very old before me. No-one has cared for it or decorated for a long time: look at the dust! At least Aggie and I know how to clean. I'm not so sure about Beth. I must get those sheets, make those curtains.

A few days later and we have moved in. I have brought Aggie over and over and shown her where she will sleep. I have brought her paper and her pencils, and her record player with all her 78s: she has a big collection of records now, mainly choral works, and she can play them and sing with them, but she also just likes to sit and watch them turning, round and round. I think she finds it calming, and certainly she seems to have accepted this move very calmly. She seems to like this room, our bedroom, and happily sleeps in her bed pushed up next to mine. She still comes into my bed at night from time to time, but not so often, and thank goodness she seems to have little interest in men now; but I still welcome her, and our lovemaking is warm and gentle and reassuring, I think. Maybe the high windows, the floor boards, and the dark old tiling remind her of the asylum.

Beth has scoured the junk shops for lengths of fabric, silky and shiny and all different colours, and she's hung them so her two rooms look like an Arabian tent. I've told her she mustn't burn her incense up there or we shall have a fire. But maybe when Lulu's a bit older we shall all sit up there and read from *Tales from the Arabian Nights*.

I thought it would be nice to have Beth here, and Lulu is a delight. I asked Ramesh to help me draw up a "contract" for Beth. I felt we both needed to be clear about our relationship: I fear she is a bit of a 'fly-by-night'. She lives here in exchange for keeping house and looking after Aggie; while we look after Lulu, so she has time to go out and to do her writing. Aggie and I like to light the fire in the evening and sit by it listening to the wireless and playing with Lulu. I am budgeting to buy a television, but that will have to wait, as there are so many other things we need, like carpets and a dining table, and most of all a new cooker.

Lulu is learning to walk. She pulls herself up on the furniture to stand and then she will let go and balance for a few seconds before she sits back down with a bump. It makes me laugh. But the other day, as she was balancing there, Aggie put her hand out and offered Lulu a finger to hold. You know, I've never seen her do anything like that before: Aggie generally doesn't seem to understand or be able to predict other people's needs, or wish to respond to them, but she let Lulu grab hold of her finger and she didn't take her hand away until Lulu let go.

Aggie really seems to like the baby. I was worried that having Lulu live with us might upset her, but Aggie seems fascinated by her. She will sit quite immobile and watch her, if she's asleep or playing quietly, for a long time. Sometimes Lulu's crying upsets her, and she'll put her hands over her ears, and sometimes she'll start screaming as well, which often shocks the baby into silence, or makes her cry even more, of course, but mostly Aggie seems to accept her infant unpredictability.

On occasions Lulu will crawl across the floor to her and pull herself upright on Aggie's skirts (Aggie still wears long skirts by preference, which are good for pulling yourself up on), and Aggie never objects, though she still will not tolerate anyone else touching her. I wonder what will happen as Lulu grows up. I think maybe Lulu is teaching Aggie, in a funny sort of way, about how people and relationships "work". Maybe... I hope... but we shall see.

II

B ETH IS A MYSTERY TO ME! I DON'T KNOW
where she goes in the evenings, and she rarely brings
anyone back here. She wears such strange mixtures of
clothes, skirts that are either very short or very long, and jeans,
or flared trousers. And brightly coloured woolly jumpers with
thick rolled necks. She says she's joined the Women's Liberation
Movement, a bit like Liza, I suppose, what was it she was a
member of? The WSPU? I think she was a suffragette, but
we've all got the vote now. Beth seems to think women have
still got rights they need to fight for, though.

Tonight she should be home. She went off two days ago, said
she was going to Birmingham and would be back today. Aggie
and I don't mind; we like looking after Lulu. But she should be
back when she promises: we've kept Lulu up to see her.

There, I can hear her key in the door.

"Oh, Mary, I'm so sorry I'm late. Where's Lulu? Let
Mummy hug you. Mary, it's been so exciting: I've been to the
Battle of Saltley Gate, that's what they're calling it. I joined the
pickets."

I get up to clear the bricks from the floor before they trip someone, and Lulu looks wistfully down at them. She was enjoying building towers with Aggie. I am cross. I've heard about this on the news. Something to do with strike-breaking lorry drivers taking the coal from the coke plant in Birmingham. I don't begrudge the miners their support. I remember the sirens and the pit collapse when I was working in the kitchen at the hospital. It's dangerous and dirty work. They deserve their money. But I don't see why Beth has to get involved: she's a mother after all.

Her face is flushed and she talks very fast. "Mary, it was so exciting. There were miners from all over, Wales, Yorkshire, come to join the picket lines. Arthur Scargill, he's from Yorkshire, stood on the roof of a public loo to tell us the Battle of Saltley Gate would go down in history. I joined the pickets and we were shouting, *close the gates, close the gates*. Because it wasn't fair. The miners just wanted a living wage and the scab lorry drivers were getting paid much more 'an them."

"Why are you so angry?"

"Why shouldn't I be? The government has no right to do this, to oppress the working men. Other union men, and women, came to support the miners. It was when the men from the Rover plant came marching over the hill with their banners and all that the police and the scabs backed off and we knew we'd won."

"Well, I've had to stock up on candles for when the electricity goes off."

"Isn't that a small price to pay for workers' rights? Come here, Lulu, and give your mummy a cuddle. One day you'll understand why we have to fight the bastards. You and me, one day we'll do it together, just us against the world. And, you know what, we'll win."

Lulu wriggles in her arms and whimpers.

"It's past her bedtime, Beth, she's tired. We kept her up to see you."

I am grumpy, but suddenly Beth is contrite. "I know, but I'm not a bad mother. I'm glad you kept her up, but she'll fall asleep here in a minute, and I don't want to let her go. I do love her so, but sometimes I have to go away. And I know she loves you, and dear Aggie. And when I'm here I look after her well, don't I?"

Lulu's eyes have closed, and her thumb is in her mouth. Beth moves to the sofa and cuddles up to me. I have been unsettled since she blew in through the front door, dropping her duffel coat and her rucksack on the floor as she came. I stroke the top of her head. Her fair hair is plaited into a thin little pigtail, and looks as if it could do with a wash. I think we all need to calm down again, except Aggie, who seems unperturbed by all the excitement. I feel I need to be reassuring.

"No-one has ever said you're a bad mother, Beth."

But then, "Anyway, I'm expecting another baby." She pulls away from me, all contrition gone, and looks me straight in the eye as if she's daring me to be angry.

I *am* angry, and I'm shocked. To have one baby out of wedlock is sad, I know that, but to have two bastard children… that's not fair. That's not fair on me, or the children. And yet, I think Ramesh predicted this. There was something in the way that he wrote that contract for Beth. But now I stand up. All I can think of to say is, "When?"

I want to shake her. I want to cry. I thought I had everything under control here. What right has she to upset everything? I lost my baby. She has hers. I was helping her to do all the things I couldn't do, and now she's throwing it all back in my face. I stand up and walk to the window. It's not quite dark outside: a half-moon, high in the sky, is fighting a losing battle with the electric light from our window to illuminate the path to my front door.

"I'm three months now. I've been to the doctor."

"But why? You've got one baby, and I thought you wanted to be a writer. And you've got a job here. I think you could have thought…"

"Oh, Mary. I love being pregnant. I love having this little thing growing inside me. I love creating something that will love *me*. And anyway, I want Lulu to have a brother or sister. I never did, and maybe things would have been different if I had."

"So have you told your parents?"

"Why should I? They've never shown any interest in Lulu."

She was right, I suppose. Her mother had visited once since we lived in this house. She had stayed for a cup of tea and hardly spoken to Lulu. When she left there were awkward goodbyes as Beth fussed with Lulu and avoided any physical contact with her. I had never met her father; he had not visited at all, and, as far as I was aware, Beth had never been to see him since she had lived with me. Not that long, really, but if she'd been my child I'd have wanted to know where she was living and with whom.

"You know, they never told me I was adopted till I was thirteen. And then they only said that I was *illegitimate*, as if that were the worst thing in the world, and that my mother had died not long after I was born. I was being bullied at school. This girl kept telling me I didn't look like my mum or dad and I must be a gypsy child. I got into a fight with her, went home with scratches on my face and my hair all messed. My shirt had got torn and my dad was furious at having to spend more money on my school uniform. I was so angry. He never showed me any sympathy when things went wrong at school, so I shouted at him that perhaps I wasn't his anyway. So he just said, too right, pity we ever picked you. And I screamed back, then why did you? And stormed out of the room. And he shouted after me, 'Bastard.'"

"But they cared for you from when you were a baby."

"That doesn't mean they loved me, or that I owe them anything."

"But surely they must have loved you."

"Not my father. I was never good enough for him. Always second best. Whenever I tried to please him he'd put me down, tell me I was useless, a waste of space. He used to hit me sometimes as well. Not often, but one day we were having breakfast when my mum complained about her hair. I said, just joking, *you should get it dyed, go blonde, but you haven't got the nerve.* It was only a joke, but he called it insubordination, and he took his belt off and thrashed me. It was after that I started staying out at night and I met Mark and he was kind to me so I let him fuck me."

"But didn't your mum love you?"

She sighs. "I think she probably did, 'specially when I was little. I can remember cuddling up to her when she read to me. She was very good at reading stories. We loved the *Just So Stories*, and later *The Secret Garden*, and *The Eagle of the Ninth*.

"But he always came first. She would never stand up for me. If I wanted to go to a party, or I wanted to wear something, and he said no, she would never support me. If he was shouting at me or sneering at me for something I'd done she would never defend me.

"I hated her for that. I still hate her. I can't forgive her. Aren't mothers supposed to protect their children whatever? She betrayed me." She is sobbing now and I sit down beside her on the sofa again and put my arm round her. She shrugs it off.

"Perhaps she was frightened of him."

"I don't care. I don't care. It wasn't right. She didn't love me enough." And she stands up and walks out of the room, carrying Lulu, still asleep, in her arms.

In a little while I follow her up the stairs, but her door is closed and she doesn't answer my knocking. Perhaps we're not that different. They called me a moral defective, she was called a waste of space, but she's fighting back. I let myself be drowned. And yet... I'm still angry with her. I have befriended her. I deserve a bit of consideration, well, more than she has given me, anyway, I think.

III

WHEN I SEE BETH next it is breakfast time. Lulu is in her high chair smashing a soft-boiled egg that has been opened out onto a piece of toast, with her plastic spoon. She has golden splashes of egg yolk on her face and her tray, and is clearly delighted with the mess she's making. She squeals with pleasure as Aggie follows me into the kitchen. Beth says good morning, but then there is a frosty silence between us. She is obviously not going to apologise and neither am I.

But I smile as I watch Lulu in her chair and I remember how she reaches out to me to be picked up from her cot when she wakes and Beth is not there, and my heart misses a beat as I realise how much I'd miss her if she weren't there.

Suddenly Beth turns to me. She looks fearful. "You won't throw me out, will you? Mary, I can still do my work for you, and look after Aggie when you need me to."

I hesitate. "Of course not, but you must think hard about the future and how you are going to support two children, and we must talk to Ramesh again about your contract."

"I know. I won't let you down. I know I'm lucky to be here."

"So you should. I had one baby and they put me in a lunatic asylum. You are going to be blessed with two, so don't behave like a spoilt child yourself."

I think we have called a sort of truce, but it still feels as if a barrier has grown between us. I think it will need Priya or Leah, both skilled moderators, to pour oil on these troubled waters. They are often here, Priya during the day, when Ania and Paul are at school and she is not at work (she works in the old mental hospital again), and Leah in the evenings.

I still don't have a lot of furniture, but my house is cosy. I have a carpet or two and bean bags to sit on. And I have a beautiful new cooker, my first really expensive purchase for my home, so there is always good food to eat: those little Jewish pastries I always wanted to make, gingerbread men for the children, filled pies for Ramesh, Priya's samosas and ladoos.

I had hoped that Leah would help Beth with her writing, and she has. They often sit together on the floor in my little front room, their heads almost touching as they read something, or argue about the best way of saying something. They are so alike they might be sisters. They both have that fine sandy hair, a bit like mine, but mine is going grey now. Leah is much taller, and, of course, she has that lovely Canadian accent. It's a bit exotic. Reminds me of those Westerns on the television: I still can't tell the difference between American and Canadian.

Beth wants to write a novel for children, a novel about a child who has been adopted. I think it must be her own story, but the bits that I hear are positive and funny. Leah keeps telling her she must make things happen to "show" her story, not just "tell" it.

"But there's a bit missing," Beth says one day, while she and Leah are playing with Lulu on the floor.

"What's that?"

"Her birth mother. Wouldn't she want to know about her birth mother?"

"Do you?" Leah asks.

"Oh yes, and I've tried to find out. I know the adoption agency that placed me. My mother let that slip when they told me I was adopted, so I went to see them. They said they couldn't help me, that women who placed children for adoption were guaranteed secrecy. But I said my birth mother had died, and they said that made no difference: there might be other relatives who might be affected if the truth came out. So I asked if the children didn't have any rights... and they said: no! Can you believe that?"

"Oh yes, that's easy to believe... this is the country that sent thousands of children abroad, to Australia, Canada, South Africa... and lied to them and their families about what would happen to them." I've never heard Leah sound bitter like that. She writes beautiful poetry herself. Beth and I both like to hear her read it out aloud to us. Much of it is about women and their struggles, so I can see why Beth likes it... some of it is quite angry, but not bitter like this. Most of her poems are tender and warm and even funny, especially when she writes about the farming folk she grew up with in Alberta in Canada.

"Do you know, though, my mother came from this part of the world, back in the 1920s. She was orphaned by the Spanish 'flu. She was sent out to Canada by one of the big children's charities. To the prairie lands and the sunshine of beautiful Alberta! Sounds like an advertisement, doesn't it?"

"My brothers were sent to Canada from the Children's Village."

"There were thousands of children sent. Said to be orphans, but many of them weren't. Do you know where your brothers went?"

"No, we never heard anything more of them." It's not often I think of Tommy and Sam these days.

"My mother couldn't, or wouldn't, remember much about her life before Canada. Her first memories were of living with a big group of boys and girls in a bunkhouse on a farm, though she thought she could remember the journey by ship that took her there. The British Home Children, they were called. She always says she wasn't badly treated, but they had to work hard in return for their food and lodging and for a minimum of schooling, and they were beaten if they fell out of line. And one day she was punished for peeling the potatoes too thickly and made to eat the peelings for her tea. She used to laugh about things like that, but I think those memories hurt."

"Do you think that's what happened to Tommy and Sam, my brothers?"

"Who knows? Some of the children were more formally fostered or adopted, but many were just treated as cheap labour. It all depended where you were sent. Many were ashamed of feeling like beggars and just wanted to forget what had happened to them, to begin again, to make their own way in the world. And the press and even the Canadian government often didn't make them welcome. There was talk of them being drawn from the dregs of society and of this 'infecting' the Canadian character."

"What happened to your mother?"

"She worked for the farmer's wife, cleaning and washing and doing chores like that, until they didn't want her anymore and sent her back to the charity that had placed her. Then they helped her get a job of her own in service, and she started to earn some money of her own. She was pretty and she liked dancing. She married a 'true' Canadian, a farmer's son she met at a dance. Over time she just 'forgot' her British roots. I think the hurt of being abandoned by her home and her family and sent away was just too much for her."

"So you didn't come to find them?"

"No, I wasn't interested. I don't feel drawn to anything here. I made a few enquiries, Ramesh helped me, but I didn't try very hard. I did find the orphanage she was sent from and that did confirm that she *was* an orphan, unlike many that were 'transported'. But I belong in Canada. I came to England out of a wider curiosity. I wanted to travel the world. I could get a job here quite easily to start off."

"Maybe that's the way my brothers think; they're Canadians now."

"Many do. England is a world away, in distance, in their timeline, in financial commitment."

"But they must feel some sort of tie… if they had a sister…"

"Perhaps it's their children or their children's children will feel the tie, or perhaps the tie is just too painful to recall, best suppressed."

"No, I can't understand that," Beth chips in. "Don't people need to know where they come from? Isn't it part of who they are? Don't they need to belong somewhere?"

"You can create a new life, a new belonging. You can live in the present and not in the past. Regret is so destructive: it makes you angry. And being angry poisons your happiness. I know. Don't forget I lost my baby; I lived in an asylum."

"But that was a long time ago." She is quite dismissive.

"Beth, that is so unkind. And what about your children? Will they know who their fathers were? Have you told their fathers that they may have children? Don't they have a right to know?"

"That's different. Lulu is loved; she, and the new baby, they won't need to know who their fathers were. They'll have me. Always. And they'll always be loved. I can tell them everything they'll need to know about their fathers."

"No, Beth. Listen to yourself. I still think they may want to know about their fathers, out of curiosity. You're talking about knowing where you come from, and denying *them* that. Love isn't everything. And shouldn't their fathers know them? Aren't you denying them *their* right to know their own children?"

She ignores me. Lulu is building a tower of bricks. They both scream as it topples and falls to the ground.

"This is my life, and my children. Don't dictate to me, Mary. I don't see that you've tried to find your child's father. Or perhaps you never knew who the father was?"

I am astounded. I feel as if she's slapped me hard across the face, like the nurses sometimes did if you stepped out of line in the asylum. I can't breathe. She picks up Lulu and walks out of the room, slamming the door shut as she goes.

Leah looks uncomfortable. "Sorry, Mary, I shouldn't have started that discussion. Understanding who you are and where you come from is such a complex thing."

All I know is Beth and I have fallen out again, and once more the foundations of my "safe house" are crumbling. And is she right? Did I never give a thought to the father of my child? Did James have the right to know he was a father? Should he have known about Peter? How could he? I was locked up in a mental hospital. But Molly knew and she didn't tell him. Until he was dying. But I could have found him; that wouldn't really have been so very difficult. I never tried. I never thought to.

IV

Once more Beth and I are hardly speaking to each other. I confide in Priya. We sit in my back room and do our yoga together.

"You must remember she is very young."

"Like I was when I first went into the asylum? No, Priya, she is not a baby. She is selfish and unkind."

"Be patient with her. She feels she is not loved. And she still has to grow up. And you, Mary. You cannot expect her to make the 'belonging' you want of her. You cannot use her to create the home, the family you search for. That is not fair on her."

"Perhaps."

"Mary, I have told you before. The asylum was part of who you are. There is only one person who can help with your 'belonging'. I feel it inside me. You should find her again. I know she is, how you say, 'uncomfortable' to be with, I know she has made mistakes, I know she has hurt you, but she has known you longer than anyone, except for maybe Aggie. She is the only person who can bear witness to your history, to who you really are."

"You mean Molly?"

"Of course. Now let go of your anger. Look beyond it. Hear the wind."

But I am not in the mood for distraction. "What about *your* 'belonging', Priya?" I challenge her. If she can challenge me I can get my own back. But she disarms me.

"I think I am growing to love Ramesh, Mary." She laughs and her face goes red. "I think I must thank you. You made him see I was not just an ignorant woman. You made him respect me."

"Not me. Look at you, you were so strong. You went on being yourself when he would have turned you into an English wife, or what he thought was an English wife."

"But he has made my children English and I am sad. And I think he will be sad too. There is a temple, a Hindu temple, in town and we have visited. Our community is growing. It is where we are beginning to belong. We can still be British and not forget where we came from. He will see that one day.

"He has had a bad life. He does not talk of it. But it has made him so he does not trust people. He wants to be close but he doesn't know how. He is very, how you say, mixed up. I think he needs to learn he can trust me. He needs to know if I am strong he is still safe. We can be, how is it, partners.

"I will tell you, but you must keep secret. His family lived in Lahore when he was a boy. Before the British left India and it was divided into Pakistan and Hindustan there was much fighting and his family left for Delhi. He saw things a young man should not see: cruelty and killing and torture, friends turning into enemies, his father begging for his life, his mother in a refugee camp, poor and hungry. That is why he talks always of assimilation. Difference, as he thinks, means anger. Sometimes, even now, he has terrible dreams."

"What happened to them then?"

"His family had relatives in Gwalior. They escaped the camps in Delhi and came there. They lost all their property, but Ramesh's father was a clever man, and his mother sewed some of her jewels into her clothes, so they made a new business and money to send their boys to school and college. So Ramesh did well, and came to UK. Oh, but married me first!

"And he is a funny man, and I like that. I am learning to make joke of him. How you say, tease him, and he likes that."

"He likes the ladies, Priya."

"I know that. I got angry but he promised he would never be disrespectful of them or of me, so now I just watch and I tease him. And I tell him he looks like a big baby when he plays up to them."

"Oh Priya, sometimes *you* are so funny. But tell me about the hospital. What's it like now?" I feel better. I have forgotten Beth's hurtful words.

"Well, they have closed a lot of the wards, though there are still some left with 'long-stay' patients on them. They are trying to move them out as well. But they are using some of the old front wards for more – what they say – 'acute' cases, that are there for short times for treatment. There are more medicines for them now, though they still use the electric shocks."

"Have they stopped the operations now though? I hope so, the – what did they call them – the lobotomies, that used to turn the patients into 'zombies.'"

"They don't do any operations in the hospital now. And they try to send the patients to the district general hospital when they can."

"Ah yes, to a mental ward in a 'real hospital', as Molly would have said."

"Some of the old buildings have been made for use as clinics or day units. There's even one unit for young people, not children but not grown yet. But, Mary, they still use the old kitchens."

"The 'long-stay' patients are all getting old now. I see them sometimes in the village, buying their cigs or drinking tea in the Best Breakfast Café: that's the only one that really welcomes them. But I think the meals will not be as good now, even if they use the kitchens. They haven't got the farm to supply the meat and veg now. I know that's gone. But do you like working there, Priya?"

"I like to work. And I like the patients. I didn't used to, but then the patients didn't like me. Now they know me, and we are friends. Come, you will not concentrate on yoga. Let us go and make chai."

In the kitchen Beth is feeding Lulu. She does not speak to me.

"Have you found about your mother yet, Beth?"

"A bit, Priya. I went back to see my adoptive mother again, and, of course, she had stuff she'd never told me about, like a postcard to me from my real mother."

"What did it say?"

"Just that she loved me but she couldn't care for me because she was too ill, but she hoped I would be happy. It was just a scribbled note in pencil, but it was signed Lydia Rose, so I know her Christian names. And it was addressed to Elizabeth, so I know she gave me my name. And I've mithered the adoption agency. They won't give me information, but they said if I had specific questions they would try and answer them. So I know she died of TB, and I know she was Irish, and I know she was Catholic, though that was obvious: after all, I was placed by a Catholic agency."

"So what do you do now?"

"I think maybe I can find where she died: I know when. And maybe that will give me her full name. Leah's helping me. She's been doing some searching herself."

I thought Leah wasn't interested in chasing her "roots". I feel excluded. Why won't they talk to *me* about these things?

V

I HAVE HEARD RAMESH'S HISTORY BUT I'VE NOT REALLY
heard Priya's. Sometimes when Priya is working I collect
her children from school and bring them here for tea.
They like to play together in the garden, though Paul is
obsessed with football, and I fear for my roses, so I often
take them out into the park across the road. If they are too
noisy and boisterous it sends Aggie to our bedroom to watch
her 78s going round and round, and to listen to her music.
They make me realise that I am growing old, but I am so glad
I have them around me; this is what I wanted from Beth and
Lulu.

Paul and Ania are testaments to the "assimilation" strategy.
They are truly English, as their father wanted. They look
English, they speak without their parents' accent, they take
part in all the customs and festivities their friends enjoy,
particularly at Christmas, and they eat English food. Their
mother still celebrates the Hindu festivals but only in a very
quiet way, often just with me, and they are not growing up
knowing or understanding the culture they were born into.

This is very sad, but I think it may change. You surely don't need to lose your identity to belong.

I worry about Priya, though. She still wears saris, and bangles on her arms, and doesn't eat meat, and I can see she would love to include her children in the rituals that are still so important to her. She has taught me how to wear a sari, and taken me to her temple, which is in fact an old vacated community centre; and one day she says she will take me to celebrate Diwali there.

She talks to me now a lot about her family in India. She would like to see them again. Occasionally she has news from her sisters, written in characters I can't decipher on a flimsy blue airmail letter sealed round the edges with glue. And from time to time she replies, but I think these communications only make the distance seem greater.

"Gwalior, my home, is a big city," she tells us. It is school time, so Ania and Paul are not here, but Priya and Leah are not working today. "My father worked for the government offices, and we were not poor. But I have many sisters and my father was glad when my marriage was arranged. If I hadn't come to England I would have had to move to live with Ramesh's family, which would have felt almost as far away from my sisters as England!" She laughs.

We are sitting on the floor winding wool into balls from long skeins. Priya and Aggie and I are crocheting "granny" squares to make into blankets for the children. The colours are bright, greens and browns, white and yellow: spring colours of celandines and snowdrops bursting through newly green grass among the still-bare trees. The blankets will bring the garden into their bedrooms. The colours are very "English", not the colours Priya normally favours.

"India is on my list of places to visit," Leah says. "What's it really like, Priya?"

283

"I don't know how to say. I had never been anywhere but Gwalior before I came here. The streets there are very wide and busy, with cows wandering in the way. Often there is dust, but always there is colour and noise: spices and chillies for sale, and flowers for the temple. Sometimes the cows are painted. Off the main streets there are narrow lanes and passages and the cows get even there. Our house was quite big, on two floors with a wall outside. Outside the house there was always a paan seller, so there were always men, chewing paan and spitting, and from the top of the house you could see a river, maybe not a river but a stream, with the potter beside it making the clay cups for the chai sold to the passengers on the trains. And there were always beggars, and pigs running wild, and sometimes monkeys."

"Did you go to school?"

"Oh yes. I learnt some English and to read and write, but I had four older sisters, and by the time it came to me I think my parents were tired of educating daughters."

"But India has produced lots of clever, powerful women. I think it had something to do with Gandhi."

"My father spoke of Gandhiji. He cared for all who were downtrodden or poor, and he respected women."

"So, how did you get to England?"

"I had to wait till Ramesh sent for me. We were married before. I had to take the train, sitting in a 'ladies only' carriage, for many, many hours to Bombay. I remember there was an older woman in the carriage with me. She was wearing a pure white sari, so she was a widow. It was so hot in the carriage but she would not let me open the window. She said it would let the smuts in from the engine. She had lots of little parcels of food, which she kept unwrapping and eating one by one, and she never offered me any!

"Once I got to Bombay I was met by a cousin of Ramesh, who took me to the ship that was to bring me to Southampton."

"I came from Canada by ship as well. You can fly now but it's ever so expensive."

"I was in a cabin with three other young women, all going to join their husbands in England."

"I had to share a cabin as well, but there were only two of us."

"We slept on bunk beds in a tiny space, which was not good when we were seasick. It was best to stay on deck, but when the ship went up and down with the waves and the decks were wet with spray my shoes slipped and I fell and got wet. But then I could bathe in the great baths that the stewards filled with hot sea water, which made me feel much better. And they would leave you fresh water to rinse the salt off after. I felt like a maharani!"

"Weren't you frightened? I think it must have been really frightening for the British Home Children who came to Canada by boat." Leah looks thoughtful.

There is a ring from the door bell and Priya stands up to answer it.

She quickly comes back. "There is a very strange gentleman wants to speak with you. His dress is very untidy and I do not think he has washed. He looks like a paan seller!" She giggles.

I go to see who it is. On the doorstep is a tramp, a "gentleman of the road". His clothes are worn and torn and stained, and he is unshaven, with long dark curly hair streaked with grey that desperately needs cutting, or at least a good brush. He carries a rucksack with cups and cutlery and makeshift tools attached. I do agree with Priya that he could do with a bath.

He has gentle, grey, sad eyes, and the eyes and the hair remind me of someone.

"My name is David Atkinson. I think you may have known my mother, Ruth."

I stare at him. I cannot speak, I cannot believe what I think I am seeing.

He stands looking back at me, uncertain, almost frightened.

"Oh, my goodness, Ruth's baby," I whisper. I have no breath; I can't manage louder.

"Can I ask, do you remember her, can you tell me about her?"

Priya is clearly anxious about this strange man, now that she has stopped giggling at her own, rather weak, I fear, paan man joke; but there is no mistaking his mother's looks.

"Priya, it's fine. This young man isn't dangerous. I knew his mother. Come in, David, come and sit in the kitchen. Would you like coffee, tea? Are you hungry?"

"I didn't come for food."

"No, but you shall eat." Priya has gathered herself together again and left the paan man in Gwalior. She sets about preparing eggs and vegetables, and thick sweet chai.

"How did you find me?"

"It's a long story, but you did know my mother? And you did put up a memorial to her?"

"I did, and yes, I knew your mother, but it was a long time ago. It was when you were a baby, but I never saw you. Your mother used to talk about you though."

"Was my mother in the asylum?"

"We both were. She had what they called then melancholia, depression."

Priya hands him a mug of hot chai and he cradles it in his hands as if warming himself on it.

"Please, tell me what happened to her."

"Don't you know?"

"No. No-one spoke of her."

"But it must be forty – more – years ago. Surely, when you grew up?"

"They just said she'd been ill and died. If I asked about what she died of or where she was buried I was hushed up and told it was too painful for my father to discuss. By the time I called myself an adult it didn't seem important anymore."

"So, what happened to you?"

"When I was a baby I was looked after by my aunt, but she had children of her own. I don't remember that. But then I went back to my father and he had nannies to care for me. I didn't see much of him; he was always working. Then he married again. My stepmother was very young and beautiful, and she gave my father three more children. She didn't really know what to do with me. She never knew how to talk to me. And no-one talked about my own mother."

He pauses to drink his chai. Aggie wanders into the kitchen and walks round the table. Leah has come in too, but she quietly says goodbye and slips out. Beth has come downstairs as well, with Lulu on her hip, but busies herself getting Lulu's tea.

"You must eat omelette," Priya says.

"Thank you, this is very good." He has a deep, warm, cultured voice, and again I am reminded of Ruth.

Aggie is walking slowly round and round the table.

"This is Aggie. She knew your mother as well."

Aggie has started singing, very softly, but the tune is unmistakeable: "Dear Lord and Father of Mankind." How does she know? I feel a catch in my throat and my nose stings as the tears fill my eyes. I quickly blow my nose.

"Your mother was very beautiful. She had long, thick, black curly hair like yours, and pale skin and grey eyes. But she was just so sad she didn't want to go on living. They didn't have the treatments they have now for depression."

"Did she commit suicide?"

"I'm afraid so; she hanged herself."

"I went to look for her grave, and found her memorial, on someone else's grave."

I explain about Liza.

"The rector told me it was you did that."

"I did. But how did you come to be living this life? You look like a vagrant."

"I had my first breakdown towards the end of the war, when I was in the Forces. I was eighteen. I developed a paralysis. They said it was hysterical. I suppose I was just full of despair. I couldn't believe all the killing could be right but there was no way out of it, so my body invented a physical illness, and I got invalided out of the Army. Managed to go to university, though, after that, got a degree and worked as a teacher. I loved that, but I couldn't hack it, got depressed and had another breakdown, so I lost that job. And that kept happening after that. It just got harder and harder to find somewhere that would take me. Started owing money for my keep and things, and that's how I ended up on the road with a bottle for company.

"Actually it's not a bad life. There are routes we travel and a kind of comradeship among us tramping men. And the Sally Ann, the Salvation Army, has some good places you can put up in."

Beth is looking starry-eyed. "A real live 'Supertramp,'" she says.

"It's not that glamorous, I'm afraid, but it's not that dreadful either."

Beth introduces herself and Lulu, who hides her face from the stranger. "Did you never know about your mother, through all that time?"

"Not till I started looking for her grave. When I was ill I wondered about her, but they never told me, and I was too immersed in my own misery to think much about her."

"She loved you dearly," I tell him. "In fact her greatest sadness was that she couldn't love you enough, and her greatest fear was that she couldn't protect you from the world around you."

"I have so many questions."

"Would you like to see where she was? Priya works at the old mental hospital, and she and I, I think, could arrange that. Would it help? Or would it be too awful?"

"I would like to begin to put together some more pieces of the jigsaw. I might be able to start to understand a bit more who I am."

"And can I come too?" Beth asks. Her initial excitement at meeting this exotic stranger has disappeared. She is calmer and quieter and I think she may be realising the enormity of what has happened to this poor man.

Priya sees it's time to collect the children from school. "Our house has many rooms. I will send my husband to collect you. You will stay with us tonight, and bathe, and I will find some of Ramesh's clothes for you. Then tomorrow we will go to the hospital."

And so it is arranged. And as we wait for Ramesh, Beth feeds Lulu and listens, and he and I talk some more, about Ruth, and about Aggie and Liza and me, and he tells me more about his childhood, and the nomadic existence he now lives. There is an emptiness in his eyes, and I want to reach out and put my arms around him. I feel as if I have known him for a very long time. But we are much too polite. We sit around the table and talk of things that have happened. We never really say how we feel. I think we dare not. We are frightened of how painful it might be.

And deep in my heart is guilt. I do not want to think of how angry Ruth made me feel when she could see her baby and I could not, and how jealous I was of how close she got to Liza. I have never stopped telling myself there was nothing else I could have done.

Beth, though, leaves Lulu and goes over to David. She reaches down to him and puts her arms round him.

VI

THE FOLLOWING DAY PRIYA AND DAVID ARE on our doorstep early and we walk up to the old hospital. David is clean-shaven and wearing one of Ramesh's old suits with a roll-neck sweater under the jacket. His hair is still very long, but he looks much more respectable. He has cut and scrubbed his fingernails, which were black with dirt when he first came to my door, and he smells much better.

In the administration block we find a young lady and explain that we want to visit Ward 4. Priya tells her who we all are and she goes off to find out if it's possible. We take seats, as bidden, on the chairs in the entrance hall. I think we must look a strange sight, one Asian lady in a sari, one old biddy, a very tall upright young man with very long hair, and a heavily pregnant slip of a girl! We do not speak.

The walls around us are tiled with the same green tiles as the wards but the dark wood panelling above them shines with polish, and is edged with intricate carving. There is a vast ornate fireplace but no fire, and wide stairs lead upward to the floor above. The tiles on the floor are red and black: a mosaic of squares and triangles. There are corridors leading off from the hall, and I remember Molly's room was along one of them. This bit of the hospital hasn't changed at all.

When the young lady returns she says we may visit the ward, but a caretaker will have to accompany us. The ward has been emptied and is used now only for storage. We cannot visit the ground floor, where our day room was, as this now houses what she calls "outpatient facilities".

We wait for the caretaker. He comes jingling a set of heavy keys. I catch my breath. It's a strange feeling: they are the same keys. I cannot forget them. So many nights locked in, that last sound of the key turning.

He leads us down the corridor. This way for the ladies' wards, that for the men, and our steps echo, the way a footfall always did. We go up the stairs and he unlocks the door.

There are our old beds stacked against the walls, and everything – the beds, the floor, even the windows – is dusty. Still, the light shines through the windows, though, and the dust dances in its shafts. The tall, high windows are just the same. We stand and look. I had forgotten how vast the ward was, how high the ceiling. How many of us lived and slept, wept and dreamt, in here. It's cold and empty now. We used to warm it with our chatter, our fights, our laughter, I suppose. My legs itch at the thought of the heavy, scratchy, woollen skirts we used to put on in here in the morning for our work.

"And they locked a young woman who'd just had a baby in here?" David breaks the silence. His voice is trembling.

I remembered Ruth pacing the floor at night. Up and down, up and down.

"Is this where she died?"

How can I tell him?

But he wants to know. "She hanged herself from the metal lintel over the door there, with her bed sheet."

He walks to the door and puts his hand on the wood surround. I cannot comfort him; it's too painful for me.

Priya doesn't move. The caretaker runs his finger along the top of the tiling and blows the dust away. I am glad I haven't brought Aggie; she would have been too distressed. Beth stands drinking it all in; she looks very small in the vast room, as I must have done all those years ago.

David and I wander down the length of the ward, each in our own world. I peer through the door into the bathrooms: the old deep square sinks with their solid old-fashioned taps are still there. I expect the baths are still there as well, but I'm not going to find out.

"There used to be a table at the end here. When your mother was here there were always flowers on it, daffodils in the spring and chrysanthemums from the hothouses in the autumn.

"They used to put the flowers in heavy ceramic vases that were difficult to break. But there was one lady who always used to eat the blooms. They said she was mad, but she said that one day they'd be poisonous and she'd get ill and they'd have to take her out of here."

"Did you have no privacy?" asks Beth, her eyes wide.

"Not much, but there are worse things," I answer.

"I have been so long on the road I cannot sleep in a room without the door open now. I cannot imagine what it must have been like to be locked in here every night. Were you not frightened?"

"No, it felt safe. Even for your mother I think it felt safe." We walk back up the ward. "My bed were always just here.

"Shall we go?"

Back home David asks me more about our day-to-day life in the hospital. He finally asks why I was there, and doesn't even seem surprised at my answer. And he asks about Aggie.

"I think her family must have been told to leave her in the hospital and forget her. I think they believed then that that was best for everyone. Certainly we knew she was loved and cared for before she joined us, but her family never came to see her." Should I have tried to find them when we moved here? Would they have "owned" her? She is "mine" now, after all. And her parents will surely be dead now. Though I suppose she may have brothers and sisters.

"Aggie belongs here now. We are her family." I am surprised: Beth sounds very defensive. Does she really care about Aggie, or is this just another battle?

David stays with Ramesh and Priya for a week. Priya cuts his hair and he goes to visit his family, but then he tells us he must leave. He will take to the road again. I ask him why, and he says he prefers to be on his own now when the "demons" come to torment him. I wish I could be more helpful to him, but I think all those years of being locked away have done things to me, and I cannot reach out to him, I cannot touch him, even though I want to. I dare not. I am lying awake at night, I can hear Liza keening, I can hear my baby crying, I can hear the echo of Ruth's footfall, up and down, up and down the ward, going on for ever and ever and ever. His mother's death casts a long, long shadow.

I manage brightly, "Come back and see us again." And then I do it: I reach out and hug him tight, and suddenly we are both crying, and he is holding me tight as well, and I wish... but I'm not sure what I wish. Just that Ruth had never died, I suppose.

And then he's gone.

VII

I think BETH MUST BE GETTING NEAR HER TIME. HER "bump" is very big, but she looks so well and happy. Her hair has thickened up, like I remember mine doing. But she doesn't talk to me much. She is still quite distant. I can't think what I said to upset her so much, but then I haven't really forgiven her myself. I still think she's been very selfish.

Her main confidant is Leah. They sit up in her rooms together for hours, and then they go out together and leave Lulu with me. I insist Leah smokes her cigarettes outside: I don't want my house smelling of cigarette smoke. So they'll wander over into the park and sit on a bench together.

When I ask what they've been doing Beth says, "Leah's helping me find out about my mother."

Sometimes they will join us, me and Aggie and Priya and Ramesh, in my little front room, sitting together on the floor, but Beth's circumspection seems to have infected the way Leah talks with me as well.

Today I have lit the fire and made sticky buns for everyone to eat. Ania and Paul have been put to sleep in Aggie's and my beds (though from the stairs I can hear them talking and giggling together), and Aggie and I are making more granny squares as we talk.

"So your mother was Irish, Beth, but came to England to work?" Ramesh asks.

"It seems like it," Beth replies. "There's a big Irish community in Manchester; maybe she had ties there. She was living alone in a rented room when she gave birth to me, and when she died, though."

"The neighbour you found who remembered her, remembered a young man who used to visit; that must have been your father," Leah offers. "He doesn't seem to have been Irish."

Beth grimaces. "I can't find anything about him at all. It's so frustrating."

"Perhaps he was already married."

"Maybe…" That doesn't upset Beth. "Now I need an address in Ireland, though, for my mother. That's my first priority."

"There's an Irish association in Manchester, the Chorlton Irish Club. It was only formed in 1956, so too late for your mother," Leah says. "But a lot of Canadians trying to chase their roots make contact with it. Sometimes people remember things."

"If she had family in Manchester. They say half the nurses in the Manchester hospitals were Irish just after the war. Worth a try."

"Someone once told me there was a bar in the All Saints area of South Manchester, Auntie's Bar, which was like a sort of job centre for Irish migrants when they first arrived."

"What do you think she was like? I wonder what work she did. Couldn't have been a nurse: we'd have found her if she had been."

"I think she must have been a strong woman, like you."
Ramesh and Beth exchange smiles.

"Ramesh, how can you say that? How much of Beth's character is inherited and how much has been formed by her upbringing?" I have to challenge such a silly assertion.

"Well, she must have looked a little like me, anyway."

Beth stands up and starts to collect the cups and plates. I follow her into the kitchen. I am angry with her but I find it difficult to speak. I think she is flirting with Ramesh.

"Beth, why do you look at Ramesh like that?"

"Like what?"

"You know."

"No, I don't and even if I did I'm a free woman, and I know how to take care of myself. There'll be no more babies after this one, if that's your worry. This is the 1970s, don't forget, not the 1920s."

Then she goes back into the sitting room and the kitchen door slams behind her.

Sometimes I find her very cruel. I feel tears in my eyes. I stand at the sink and wash the cups up. I have no curtains on the kitchen windows yet and outside is very dark, but the room is still warm from my baking. I don't understand her, I don't know how to live with her. Hospital life was so much easier.

Leah comes into the kitchen. She looks wary of me. "Mary, I am off."

"When will we see you again?"

"I'm afraid you won't, Mary. I'm going back to Canada."
She has a cigarette between her fingers, and she's just returning the pack to her bag. She's ready to light it the minute she gets out of the front door!

"That's very sudden."

"Well, it is and it isn't. I think I need to see my family. But it's not the end of my travelling. I may be back, or I may not. Perhaps I'll try India next. Priya has really tempted me.

"I wanted to thank you, Mary, for your kindness to me, and apologise."

"What for?"

"I've written you a letter to explain. Here. Read it when I've gone. I've got to go now, I'm catching the night coach to Southampton, and a ship from there. Beth knows I'm going but she doesn't know what's in the letter, or at least not all of it."

"Take care, Mary." She hugs me quickly, and then walks down the hall and out the front door.

I open my letter.

My dear Mary,

I have decided to return to Canada.

I'm afraid I owe you an apology as I have not been entirely honest with you. I told you my mother's story, but I didn't tell you my father's. I didn't know the details until recently. It was Beth's search for her parents that made me follow up what I'd been told.

My father was informally adopted by the family who homed him when he came to Canada from the UK. He was in many ways one of the lucky ones: he and his brother were welcomed and loved by my grandparents, who were unable to have children of their own. His new family were farmers and were reasonably affluent, but my father was intensely ashamed of his origins, and he never came to terms with his feeling that he had come to the new country a beggar. There were many that would have bullied him for that, as well.

So he took my grandparents' name, and totally cut himself off from his roots. He called himself a "true"

Canadian, and despite my mother's history didn't tell her of his background. He took over the farm from my grandparents when they became too old to run it, and has lived, I think, a happy, successful and fulfilled life.

But secrets are difficult to keep in rural farming communities, so my mother found out. However, nothing was said to me until I decided to come to England. Then my mother told me more of their stories and also my father's real name. Neither of them wanted me to follow up their links with the mother country.

I do know, though, that my father was your brother Tommy. (Sadly Sam died of diphtheria a few years after arriving in Canada.) I did eventually visit the Children's Village and was allowed to see the records that identified Tom and Sam and named their mother and sister as their surviving relatives. As I indicated, I did this only when Beth was searching for her family, more out of curiosity than a desire to explore my roots. But then, of course, the pieces of the jigsaw all fell into place: my father's name, his history, your story about your brothers and the Children's Village.

But, I'm sorry, Mary. I could not tell you. The anger and sadness that my parents carried with them all their lives, the stigma they felt, and the strength that they had had to muster to overcome it and create a new life for themselves has infected me. I have no affection for "the mother country". It threw out its own children and lied to them and their parents.

Besides, I did not feel you were mine to own. You are my father's sister, not mine. I will tell my father about you when I get home, if I can. I hope he will let me, and I hope he will wish to contact you, but that is up to him. However, I did feel I needed now to get home and try to *share everything I've found out with them. I couldn't stay here any longer.*

But I couldn't leave without telling you this either. I felt I owed you that at least. I'm sorry I'm too much of a coward to tell you to your face.

With all my heart I wish you well and happy for many years to come.

Good luck with your writing. Don't give it up.

Your niece,
Leah.

P.S. And don't give up on Beth, please. She will grow up, and she needs you in the meantime. You both need each other, and the babies will need their surrogate grandmother: enjoy them,

Leah

The handwritten sheets fall to the floor. So that was Tommy's daughter. I want to know more, but she has gone. I should have known. It was the hair, just like mine, and they were Tommy's eyes, and Tommy's defiance.

I reach for the bottle of cooking sherry we keep in the cupboard. 'Tis not often I take a drink, but tonight I were ta'en for a fool. I trusted that young woman and she couldna' speak to me face. She were my flesh and blood but she didna' feel she belonged here. She denied me. Keepin' secrets. She were not fair.

VIII

I PUT LEAH OUT OF MY MIND VERY QUICKLY, AS
David's visit seems to have set something in motion, and
I need to give it my full attention. It feels as if a piece
of clockwork has been wound up and is ticking or revolving
slowly, like the ceiling fan that Aggie would watch in that first
café we used to visit, rotating, rotating, rotating. Shortly after
David leaves us to return to his nomadic existence, the vicar of
St Peter's comes to call. I don't think I've seen him since Liza's
funeral, and that's years ago. He is old and stooped now, but I
remember him as a kind man, and I am delighted to see him,
drawing him by the hand into my hall from the step outside.
I make a pot of tea and we sit in the kitchen to drink our
steaming mugs.

He asks me how I am, and whether I am happy living here,
then:

"Mary, there are a couple of people I'd like you to meet, as
I think you could help us."

I offer him a "squashed fly" biscuit. I've been addicted to
them since Molly introduced me to them, and now I've learnt

to make them myself, but I can't think that I'll have anything that will be of help to the vicar.

"The local history society has decided to record a history of our old asylum. Now it's gradually being closed down we think that it holds stories that will be lost for ever unless we act. We know the very old history of the place; that's been well researched and documented. But it's the more recent history we want to record. Godfrey is a retired historian and he is doing most of the work. He is collecting oral accounts of life in the asylum, from the First World War onward. These are mainly from staff: nurses who used to work there, gardeners, people like that. One of the people helping him is Molly Turner, who used to be Matron there. Do you remember her? She suggested you might be able to help."

"Of course I remember Molly. And I can try to help. What does he want to know?"

"They'd like to come and see you. They'll ask you some questions, but mainly they'd just like you to talk about what you remember."

"I think I can do that, though it's all a long time ago, and some things are better forgotten. And my memory's not what it used to be."

"Perhaps you could try writing something down."

"I do a bit of writing. And I've written down some of my experiences in the hospital before. I could try that again... my 'autobiography'! That would be very grand."

"We are taking photographs of all the old buildings as well, before they disappear. And Molly has quite a lot of old black-and-white photos of the hospital and the staff and even some of the patients, from when she worked there. And there's your recipe book... that's a bit of asylum history in its own right."

"I'd like to see the photographs. Have you seen the pictures in my book? They were done by one of the patients."

"We'd really like to know from you what it felt like to live there, and some of the stories of the people you knew in there. People like Ruth Atkinson, and Liza, whose funeral you organised. I understand she was a very interesting character."

"She was my friend. She wasn't just an 'interesting character'!"

"I'm sorry; I didn't mean to condescend or to belittle her."

"They can come and see me, but first I want to see what I can put together from the bits and pieces I've written over the years. I've kept a journal on and off as well, started it when I was learning to read and write. So that'll help."

I tell this to Priya when she visits. We sit on the floor in my back room after we've done our yoga. "Why are they so curious, Priya?"

"Is it not good that they should learn from the past?"

"What can they learn? That you shouldn't lock women up for having a baby, or being depressed? Surely they need to learn new things now. How to help them in this day and age, not what not to do."

"But it is right, is it not? That all those ladies you knew deserve to be remembered."

"Yes, you're right."

"And I have said to you before. You need to remember them; you need to talk with Molly. You cannot belong anywhere without this part of you. I saw your eyes when we visited the ward with David. That was your home."

"Mebbe."

But when she phones I do invite her to visit me. Molly... my nemesis or my archangel?

I will not be cowed by her. I sit her in my front room.

"You have a nice place here, Mary."

"Are you still living where I came to visit you?"

"Yes. It suits me. I've never had a proper home of my own, always lived in 'rooms' of one sort or another. It might have been different if my brother had lived."

There he is, James, always there between us.

"What did you want to talk to me about?"

I offer tea but she refuses.

"Three things, I suppose. Firstly: what can you tell us about your life in the hospital?"

"Probably nothing more than you can, Molly."

"Ah, but you will have a different perspective."

"I have some stuff written down and I am putting it together and writing some more."

"That will be good, but I think it might be even better if you could give us an oral account: tell your story to someone who could tape it and then write it up."

"Don't you trust my writing?"

"It's not that. I just think an oral history might be more spontaneous, and the interviewer can prompt you with questions that might be of particular interest to a new generation of mental health workers."

"Well, all right. I can do both. What was the second thing you wanted to talk about?"

"This idea of a memorial to all those that died in the hospital, the thousands of them since the asylum opened in the 1850s. We are fundraising for a plaque to be put on the wall in the church and a stone in the graveyard, and for books to contain all the names that we can find. But we need to do something to honour them all, and to mark the occasion when we put up the plaque."

"Why is this so important to you, Molly?"

"I suppose the hospital was my life. I have nothing else left now. My brother, my dear sweet little brother, is dead, and my sister's children have grown up, have families of their own, their own lives to lead. They have drifted away from me. I just have memories, and regrets. I need to do something with the thoughts that go round and round in my head, something concrete: a celebration and an expiation. Mary, I bear so much guilt and so much anger. I was a cog in the machinery that kept women like you and Liza behind locked doors."

"But that was the system."

"Ah, yes, but I believed in it. I did nothing to fight it. I even had Liza sent to Broadmoor. What for? For mourning her friend?"

"You?" The room feels cold. If I hunch my shoulders and put my hands in my armpits might I feel a bit warmer, like curling up on the floor behind my bedstead. "You? You sent her to Broadmoor? Did you hate her so much?"

"Did I? She was clever, and dangerous: all her talk of equality, respect. And you all admired her, would have followed her wherever she led, wouldn't you?"

"Yes, but you told me you didn't have the power to send her away."

"No, so I didn't. But I could influence those that did."

"So what do you want to do to honour the dead and gone?"

"I'm not sure, Mary. I think maybe we could have some sort of memorial service. What do you think? I wanted to talk to you, as I've been thinking about it ever since that day we went to the churchyard together to find those graves, and it was one reason I came to Liza's funeral."

"We could read out all the names. That way each one would have the identity they were denied while they were alive and were just another lunatic.'"

"That might be possible. I think we have found most of the names, but it would take quite a long time to read them all out. I will think about it."

"So, what's the third thing?"

The door opens and Beth flies in. She is as white as a sheet. "Mary, my waters have broken. The baby's not due for another month. What shall I do? Don't send me to the hospital. They said I could have it at home."

"But if the baby's going to be too small?"

"No, Mary, the pains have started, it's all happening too fast. Get the midwife. I've got her number somewhere. In the drawer beside my bed, I think."

"Go up to my bedroom. There's light and space in there. I'll get that number and call her. Where's Aggie?"

Molly's putting her coat on. "I'll go. You don't need me."

"No. Find Aggie. Look after her. Take her up to the top of the house. The baby's there as well. Play with them, keep them quiet."

"Me? Play with babies…"

"Aggie will show you. Lulu loves Aggie. And there's milk and biscuits in the kitchen."

I can't get through to the midwife; the line's engaged. I hang up and run up the stairs. Beth is sitting on the very edge of the bed, standing, really.

I think back to when Peter was born. "Shouldn't you lie down, Beth?"

"No." She's breathing hard. "I need to keep walking. The pain's coming again. Hold my hand, Mary." She squeezes it so hard it really hurts. "I think we need to time how often the pains are coming and how long they're lasting," she says, trying to catch her breath. "Aaaaarrrrgh… or perhaps we don't, they're coming so close. Go and try the midwife again."

I run down the stairs and dial the number again. This time there's an answer. "I'll come straight away. Call an ambulance as well, just in case: the baby may need help if it's premature."

I dial 999 before I go upstairs again. I fear Beth will tell me not to.

I can hear squeals of delight from the top of the house. Molly is obviously coping.

"Help me walk, Mary: it helps the pain." We keep walking, stopping each time the pains come, when she squeezes my hand.

"Water, pleeeaaase. I need a drink." I fetch a mug of water and a wet flannel from the bathroom, and I wipe her face. What else should I do? Blankets and towels. I fetch them from the airing cupboard.

Beth is kneeling on the floor now, between pains, sobbing into the eiderdown on my bed. "I think it's coming, Mary."

I run downstairs again and open the front door, leaving it ajar for the midwife and the ambulance men. These stairs will be the death of me!

"Oh my God, Mary. I need to push." I lift her T-shirt… the top of a head. I can see the top of a head. Beth is panting, then she takes a deep breath… and it arrives, along with two ambulance men and a midwife. I am sent away immediately to fetch hot water and a bowl (why?), and as I leave the room I hear that cry, that high-pitched, snuffly, cat-like wail that I remember so well, and I catch my breath. I am shaking and I'm crying, but I must fetch the water.

When I go back into the bedroom Beth is lying on my bed. She has the new baby in her arms and the cord has been cut but the midwife is still at work. The ambulance men have gone.

"Is she all right?"

"Mother and daughter are fine, but so much for your dates, young lady. This baby was never premature!"

Beth beckons me over and hands me the baby, wrapped in one of my towels. "Here, take her. Meet Lydia Mary, Lydia for my mother and Mary for you. Do you like her, Mary?"

She's beautiful, all messy and wrinkled but… "She's beautiful."

"Thank you, Mary, thank you for everything. That was all so wonderful. It was just beautiful bringing her into the world in this lovely room with the light shining in through these lovely high windows... just perfect. And she's just perfect. And I love you, you know. And no-one will ever take *this* little one from you, ever, Mary."

I find a little hand under the towel and it closes over my finger.

"Well, maybe. We'll see." We are both quite tearful; let's see what a new day brings. But baby Lydia Mary lies in my arms as if she were always meant to be there. I don't want to let her go, but I can send Molly home now. Whatever that third thing was she wanted to talk to me about, it will have to wait. There's supper to prepare and then some introductions to be made. What will Lulu make of her new little sister? New life begins but the old must carry on.

IX

I don't see Molly again for a while. Godfrey, the local historian, comes to see me with a tape recorder and asks me loads of questions about my life in the hospital. He tells me Molly and the vicar are planning an "event". They have collected together all the names that they can find of the men and women who died in the asylum (or later in the mental hospital), and, as Molly and I discussed, they are to have a service of remembrance when all the names are read out. They think it will need to happen over a few days, there are so many names. They want me to do some of the reading.

When my day comes I walk to the church with Aggie. There seem to be quite a lot of people coming and going, and at the back of the church there is an exhibition of pictures and plans of the old asylum. There are copies of old records, stories of patients, handwritten notes of meetings, kitchen requisitions… but all of these are very old: from long before my time, mostly from before the turn of the century. This is very old history.

It is a beautiful day. The sun is shining through the stained glass of the high window above the altar. Someone is playing the organ, gently, in the background. Aggie sits in one of the pews with a notebook, her pencil describing tiny circles swirling like bubbles blown in the wind. There is a sense of calm, but also a sense of busyness, as if we all have a common urgent purpose, to speak for the forgotten, to lay to rest uneasy ghosts, to make some sort of reparation. And then what? Turn away, forget again?

I stand and walk to the lectern. I read my list of names, slowly and clearly, so that each name can echo around the aisles, each one claiming its own identity. The names of "the mad, the bad, and the sick", each with their own story, each no doubt once loved by someone, a mother, a child, a lover... who knows. It's my final farewell to them all, and to my mother, to Ruth, to Liza.

Then I go to sit with Molly, who has found a seat in the pew with Aggie, and we listen in silence together as others read more names. Then, when the session ends, Molly turns to me. She is dressed in black, her elegant astrakhan coat unbuttoned but covering her still ample curves, a splash of red silk at her neck, her hair white and perfectly permed. I think she has dressed especially for this occasion.

"What was the third thing you wanted to talk to me about, that day Lydia was born?" I ask. Indeed, I demand. It is time she was honest with me.

"My sister." She sighs.

I soften. I take her hand. I think I know what she is going to tell me. I think I have known for a long time.

"Mary..." There is a long pause.

"James set up a trust fund for you. It wasn't in your name but he told me that it was meant for you when he was dying. It took the lawyers and the family a very long time to sort it out, but eventually you received it. I told them you weren't to know where it came from. I thought you might refuse it if you knew. Now I want you to know, because he loved you, his little sweetheart, and this is the proof.

"And I have another piece of information. May just be gossip, but possibly another piece in the jigsaw. One elderly lady whom Godfrey interviewed said she knew of a woman who had been wet nurse to a baby born to a lass who was put in the asylum. She kept the baby when her own child died and he grew up in her family, knowing her as his mother. She could have been the woman that Liza and I met. The woman Godfrey spoke to thought the baby might have died as an adult… an accident or something. The mother died not long after. But she couldn't give Godfrey any names or traceable details, though she did think the young man might have had a child. Not much to go on but…"

"Molly, he was not just *my* baby, you know. Peter would have been your nephew."

"I know. I would have liked to find him."

"Molly, you must have this." Out of my pocket I take the little black-and-white photo. "I don't need it. I remember him as the baby I held and loved. This means nowt to me; you take it."

X

S O HERE I AM ON MY SEVENTIETH BIRTHDAY. I am sitting at my desk. Lulu and Lydia came shouting into our bedroom with a tray of breakfast before they went off to school this morning, and Beth has been in and wished me "Happy Birthday", and has gone back to her room to write. We grow closer as the years pass. I think she feels that together we have created the family she would have wished for her children, the family she didn't have when she was growing up.

From my window I can see Aggie pacing the garden as she did the airing courts so many years ago. I think, in her own sweet way, she is content. The sun is shining through the window as it did through the high windows of the asylum. I have been lucky. My life has been full. I escaped the institution and, largely, its effects upon me. There must have been many who lost their babies as I did, who lost their ability to make decisions for themselves, who never escaped the asylum, who never knew what might have been. I honour their memory. I hold no grudge now against those that confined me. But I shall always keep a special place in my heart for my Peter, and I shall always wonder where he is, if he lives, and, if so, what cards life dealt him, though I am spent with searching for him.

I know, too, that Tommy made a new life for himself. He has never contacted me, but I am happy enough knowing he has lived a fulfilled life. Leah was testament to that.

Later I will see Priya. She has been my constant friend for many years now and I know how she has pined for her sisters in Gwalior. She made herself ill by not eating, but she always smiled for me. There is a growing Hindu community nearby and she goes to the temple, which seems to have given her some comfort. But what has pleased her most is that her daughter, Ania, has now started to ask about her religion and about her roots in India. And as she has reasserted this key to her identity the weight has crept back onto her hips, and the roses have reappeared in her cheeks. Even Ramesh seems more comfortable in his skin, though his return toward his own culture has not precluded lunches of steak and kidney pudding, or a whisky or two in the evening. And he no longer makes a secret of his roving eye and his admiration for the "ladies", explaining it, as he does everything now, in riddles and fractured philosophising.

This evening I shall sit where I know now that I belong: here and with Aggie. And we shall complete a jigsaw puzzle. I can't keep up with Aggie. She places the pieces by looking at the shapes, and never looks at the picture. She is so fast, and is quite happy to do the same puzzle over and over. And I will help the girls with their homework, if I can. They both like writing stories… like their mother.

Yesterday I went up to the hospital again. You can now walk freely through the walls and into the grounds. They are gradually closing it down. I have made good progress with writing the story of my time in the asylum, so I wanted to take one last look at where we lived for so long. There are a few of the wards still in use, and the administration block is still functioning, but most of the wards are now closed and boarded up, with sheets of plywood over the windows. The front of the hospital is busy with people coming and going, cars parked, neatly weeded rose beds, but no patients.

Behind, dust and discarded plastic bags blow across the airing courts, where dead-headed weeds and buddleia are the only things growing. Several of the "back wards" still have patients in them: out of sight, out of mind. I am told these are the most severely ill who are a danger to themselves or others. They have put high wire fences around them, higher than the walls and fences that kept us in. It fills even me with dread and, worse, with despair. Is this still the only way we can contain those that are different, that frighten us because we cannot understand them?

I walked up to the chapel through the grounds. The field that used to be full of chickens is no longer part of the hospital and is used by pretty little girls in jodhpurs and hard hats for keeping their ponies. The orchard has gone wild, the trees gnarled and unpruned but heavy with apples and pears. I collected some for our girls and bit into one of them... so crisp and sour. We would have stored these for the winter. The vegetable beds and the rhubarb have all disappeared, and buddleia has overwhelmed the outhouses and the remains of the greenhouses. Along the path to the cricket pavilion, now only a concrete base remaining, I found the old crab apple trees hidden in a tangle of brambles, and among the brambles some borage was growing.

I followed the path up toward the chapel. From the top of the hill I could see the winding gear above the colliery across the valley. Even that's said to be closing down soon, the sirens silenced for good, the shafts and the tunnels abandoned to the ghosts of the men who toiled there in the airless dark.

I reached the chapel. It's waiting to be demolished now. The windows have been removed and it is surrounded by welded wire panels and notices warning that it's an unsafe building. Others had been there before me and ignored the danger, so it weren't difficult to find a way through. The door was already half open.

Inside everything had been removed. There were no pews, no altar, no plaques on the walls, though curiously they'd left one small stained-glass window, high above the altar, or where the altar used to be. The sun was shining through the glass, refracted into rainbow colours, and falling as a kaleidoscope of patterns onto the far wall. They must have taken the lead from the roof so that water had come through, and weeds had germinated in the cracks between the bricks. Nature seemed to be gently and benignly reclaiming the old stones, quarried from I have no idea where, warming them with the light from the high windows, and returning them to rest with the souls of the mad, the bad, the sick or the simply unloved who had passed this way.

I sat on the cold stone floor, though I knew I should find it hard to get up again. There were cigarette ends and empty beer cans around me, sweet papers in the corners, the ashes of a fire someone had tried to light, but it were very peaceful. I remembered Aggie singing here, us on one side of the church and the men on t' other; and the doctor's wife who brought her children when the doctor had his headaches; and the texts that led us to believe that if we all prayed hard enough we would be made better. And I remembered Liza and Ruth, and the thousands of men and women who lived and often died inside the asylum walls... real people, people I cared about, people I helped to feed.

What will happen to people like that in the future? The big institutions have come and gone, meeting the needs as they were perceived then. What will be the way forward? Will we be kinder to those that follow? Kinder than we were to those we locked away? Or, if we cannot lock them away, will we leave them homeless, to wander the streets like David, seeking solace in a bottle? I hope we will have more compassion.

In my pocket was the doll. I don't know why I had brought him. I put him on a stone beside me. We had travelled a long way together, he and I, the only connection I had now with my baby. Together we watched the low sun sinking toward the horizon, and in the rustle of the breeze through the leaves on the floor I could hear again the chatter, the chink of the crockery in the dining hall, the echo of a footfall in the corridors... and mebbe yet "that still small voice of calm".

Epilogue

1953

I T IS ABSOLUTELY BLACK NOW. I CAN HEAR SOME distant muffled thumps, but otherwise it's completely silent. If I close my eyes I believe I can see some light, like shafts of sunlight through a high window, refracted into all the colours of the rainbow and dancing with silvery motes of dust. But it's just an illusion.

Earlier I could hear the sirens, but they've stopped. And I thought I could hear voices. No breath to shout them, though. I'm here, you know: don't leave me, don't forget me. And then the thumps, like the echo of a footfall...

There were thirteen of us down here, and not even miners, just the engineers sent down to survey the old tunnels, see which seams can be opened up again. Can't hear anyone else now. Must have been caught in my own air pocket. Backside's going numb and I can't move my feet, but if I reach out I can feel a section of wall. That must be a good thing, something's held up. They'll be able to follow the shaft.

Hard to breathe here, can't speak. In my pockets? A pencil, no matches, a piece of paper. I remember: my birth certificate.

Was going to show it to Rosie. Different surname. Seems me mam wasn't me mam, took me in and fed me when me real mam went into the asylum. Sort of adopted me in the place of her own baby when he died. No-one asked for me back so she sort of kept me. Never told me till I said I wanted to marry Rosie, my darling Lydia Rose. Thought I ought to know.

Rosie'll laugh. Want me to find me real mam. After the babe's born. Have to get married, after the babe and when she's well again. Then we can face her family. Never been to Ireland. Green, isn't it? The Emerald Isle? I can see waves of green light, coming from that window.

Grew up just two roads over from the asylum wall. Used to climb it for dares and scrump the apples from the orchard. They used to have cricket matches and fairs there, but Mam never let us go. Know why now.

Going to call the babe Elizabeth, if it's a girl, after the new queen. Would be married now if not for 'er cough. Had to go into hospital, lost her job and 'er wages. Couldn't afford the trip to Ireland to ask her dad. Make it okay before we go, anyway.

The colour's changed to red, more flashes than waves. Hands are warm now, were icy cold. I can hear the sea. Can't be, must be the coal face, like holding a shell to your ear. The thumping has stopped. All I can hear now is the thumping of the blood in my ears.

Rosie must get better. Get her job back. Must look after the baby if I don't get out of here.

Wonder what me real mam was like. What happened to her? Was she really mad? Did she ever want me back?

Can't breathe, face is wet… must be crying. Don't go to sleep. Must stay awake. Don't want to die. Want to find me mother… want her to see her grandchild.

Acknowledgements

THE ECHO OF A FOOTFALL IS A WORK OF fiction, although I have drawn on the many written and oral accounts of life in the old long-stay institutions, and upon my own experiences of such hospitals as a doctor in training in the 1960s and 70s. Any resemblance to real persons, alive or dead, or to events, or specific places is coincidental.

There are many people, however, to whom I am indebted for help and guidance on my journey toward the completion of this book. Thank you to you all. I would particularly like to thank Jean Tarry for getting me started on this project, for her invaluable support and advice, and for her patient reading of early drafts. Thank you, too, to Alan Kent, for sharing with me his memories of life as the child of the Master and Matron, living in a long-stay public assistance institution. My book group (you know who you are) were a constant source of inspiration through their erudite and stimulating discussions of literary form and content... thank you. And I am eternally grateful to Sue Hepworth and Mary Eminson for reading and critiquing later manuscripts. Finally, I must thank my husband, John, for his forbearance, for reading and rereading drafts, for supporting my efforts, and for walking the dog...